JADE
Forever In My Heart

THE STORY OF MY BATTLE
AGAINST CANCER

JADE

Forever in My Heart

Jade Goody

WINDSOR
PARAGON

First published 2009
by HarperCollins*Publishers*
This Large Print edition published 2009
by BBC Audiobooks Ltd
by arrangement with
HarperCollins*Publishers*

Hardcover ISBN: 978 1 408 45920 1
Softcover   ISBN: 978 1 408 45921 8

British Library Cataloguing in Publication Data available

Printed and bound in Great Britain by
CPI Antony Rowe, Chippenham and Eastbourne

Contents

Foreword

By Jackiey Budden

When my daughter Jade was born I had no idea what impact she would have on this world.

I split up with her father when she was about one and it's just been me and her ever since. Until, that is, she arrived in the *Big Brother* house and the cameras joined her.

Jade has written in her autobiographies that I was not the best mother in the world. I took drugs for four years and let her down. Before that she helped care for me after a motorcycle accident that left me severely injured and without the use of my left arm.

Jade has always been there for me. When she was diagnosed with cancer it was my chance to be a good mum—and I think I proved to her I could do it.

As a child Jade loved performing. She was always making me sit on the settee to watch her sing a song or dance. Drama was the thing she did best at school. Then she got a job as a dental nurse and focused on having the stable life she longed for.

As her mother, I was last to know she'd entered the *Big Brother* auditions until she rang me screaming, 'I've been kidnapped and am in Borehamwood somewhere!' She'd been warned not to tell anyone and because of my big mouth I wasn't told till the last minute.

Watching her on that TV screen made me so proud. Even when she stripped off for the poker game, I knew she was just trying to do the right thing. Jade was brought up to play games properly and follow the rules.

Afterwards, fame brought her more money than she'd ever imagined having. Suddenly she was able to live in a lovely house and have things she'd never dreamed of. And it didn't change her one bit. She never saw herself as a celebrity. All her friends stayed the same and she lived a normal life. Her agent at the time said this wasn't possible, but Jade proved it was.

I became a celebrity mum too and the drug days were soon behind me.

We've always had our ups and downs but this illness brought us closer than ever. Jade and I are one of the same picture. We've been best friends, flatmates, fighters, but always there for each other.

Of all her achievements, Bobby and Freddy are the ones that Jade is most proud of. They became her world and the money from her fame let her give them the life she never had.

Watching my daughter grow so ill with cancer has been a living nightmare. God has thrown some challenges at Jade and this one she tried so hard to fight for her boys.

These diaries show just how hard she fought. Despite the pain and the horrible treatments, her wicked sense of humour shines through on every page.

Jade's courage and love for her family and friends is clear for everyone to see.

I hope people feel inspired by her honesty. Jade always tells things like they are. And as her mum, I am so very proud of that.

Jackiey Budden
20th March 2009

Chapter One

The Horrible News

18th August 2008

I'd been in the Indian *Big Brother* house for three days and was really enjoying myself. They were a nice bunch of people—a famous chef, actors and actresses, dancers, even an MP—and I think I was getting on well with all of them. It was early evening and I was just on my way to the kitchen to get something to eat when the *Big Brother* voice boomed out telling me to go to the Diary Room.

Off I went, thinking they'd be giving me another task or whatever. The worst I could think would happen was that the Indian public hated me and had decided to vote me off already. I sat in the big leather chair in the Diary Room and one of the production team passed me their mobile phone.

'What's going on?' I said. 'Hello?'

It was my agent, Mark Thomas, calling from London.

'Jade,' he said, gently. 'Your consultant needs to talk to you. It's about your test results and it's very, very urgent.'

I thought it was a wind-up. 'You're kidding me?' I said. But I could tell from Mark's voice that it was something serious.

'It's potentially bad news so he's going to ring you himself,' he replied. 'Just stay there and I'll get him to give you a call.'

1

I knew straight away what it must be about. I'd had ongoing problems with my periods for years by this stage, then on the 2nd of August, a Saturday night, I collapsed at home bleeding really heavily. I called an ambulance and they took me to Harlow Hospital.

No-one knew what was wrong and they kept me in for days doing loads of tests.

I had blood tests and a scan and they all came up clear.

Then on the Wednesday they did some laser surgery. I've had this done twice before, so I knew what to expect. It's still not nice, though, I'm telling you!

Then I got a call on the Thursday from Mark.

'Guess what?' he says. 'Indian *Big Brother* want you in the house!'

I was well excited. And Shilpa Shetty was hosting it, a real sign of how things had turned around for me. But of course Mark was worried about my health.

'Make sure the docs say you're okay to do it,' he said.

I told them I'd need to be away for three months and they said it was fine. 'Take some painkillers and don't worry,' they said. I had a few more test results still to come back but no one seemed worried about them.

*   *   *

Sitting there in the *Big Brother* house waiting for the phone call, I realised it must be to do with that. It's the only health problem I had. What on earth had they found now?

2

I had to wait a whole half hour. I just sat there, fidgeting, wondering if this was a weird joke. *Big Brother* sometimes plays tricks on you—it's part of what you sign up for—but I didn't think they would do something like this. Could it be someone from home playing a practical joke? If it was, what a horrible one!

Finally the mobile phone rang again and the production assistant handed it to me.

A doctor came on the phone and introduced himself, then he launched straight in with the news.

'Jade, we've looked at your biopsy and there are severe abnormalities. You need to fly home immediately,' he said.

'You what?!' I replied.

'You have cancer, Jade. It's real and it's serious.'

He carried on talking but I couldn't hear anything any more. There was a buzzing in my ears. My legs turned to mush and I started crying. Really crying. I sank down onto the carpet.

The only thought in my head was, *'My boys! Oh my god, I'm going to die.'* I just heard the word 'cancer' and thought 'this is it!'

My tummy felt so sick, I thought I was going to throw up all over the floor.

'Are you sure?' I asked, and he told me again I needed to get myself home. That I needed treatment. That it was urgent.

When he hung up I sat there feeling lonelier than I've ever felt in my life. I was in Mumbai, in a house full of strangers, and had just been told the most horrible news. I was a million miles away from my home and everyone I loved.

It was only then that I remembered I was on a

TV programme. It's not the normal way to be told you have cancer. But then, what is normal in my life? To be honest, that seemed like the least of my worries at the time.

Someone pushed the phone into my hand and I spoke to my agent again.

'Jade, you'll be okay, love,' he said, trying to calm me down.

'I can't believe this, Mark,' I sobbed. 'Is it some kind of sick wind-up?'

'No,' he replied. 'I've checked the doctor out and he has treated you in Harlow before. I asked him if it was life or death and he said yes, you had to be told. You need to come home and we'll get a second opinion straight away.'

I just couldn't stop sobbing. So many thoughts were rushing in. I had no control.

My boys! My mum! Jack! I can't die! I don't want to, I've got too much to live for. Oh my god . . .

Cancer equalled death to me. *I'm only twenty-seven, this can't be happening.*

I tried to dry my eyes with bits of tissue someone gave me.

'Don't tell anyone until I've had a chance to let your family know,' said Mark. 'I'll call your mum and Jack as soon as we get off the line. Do you want to leave straight away? Or are you able to go back into the house and get your things?'

'I'm okay,' I sobbed. 'I'll go back in. Will you check up on that doctor again? And get a second opinion for me?'

*   *   *

Being on *Bigg Boss*, the Indian *Big Brother*, was

4

supposed to be my Big Comeback—my way of getting over all that controversy two years before when I went on *Celebrity Big Brother* and had a falling out with Bollywood star Shilpa Shetty, so it had seemed like a great idea. The money was good and I needed it because I had spent the last year living off my savings.

I never expected to win or anything but I'd wanted the people of India to see what I was really like. It wasn't supposed to end like this.

Things other doctors had told me were running through my head. They'd said they thought the heavy bleeding I'd had was just a bad period. Or stress. How could it be cancer? How could no one have seen this? How long had this cancer thing been growing silently inside of me? My whole body was shaking with fear.

I was more scared than I'd ever been in my life.

I left the Diary Room and went back into the house. I was planning to get my clothes and stuff but I could hardly see because of my swollen red eyes.

The other contestants knew straight away something was wrong. It was pretty obvious because I was sobbing so much. I went and sat on the sofa, trying to take it in.

They tried to comfort me, being really nice. Someone brought me a glass of water and someone else found some tissues, but I was in my own bubble.

I said over and over: 'I can't tell you until I tell my family first.'

But you know me—I can't keep anything to myself. Even this. Eventually I caved in and told them.

5

'I've got cancer!' I cried, the words sounding strange. Everyone was really shocked. I went to the bedroom, and just sobbed and sobbed.

I've got cancer.

I got my things together somehow then I was taken to a side door and shown out by the production team. I hardly had any time to say goodbye to the other contestants. I was just rushed away.

A car took me to a hotel somewhere. I spent the night on my own, constantly on the phone trying to ring people. I was on the other side of the world and I needed my friends and loved ones so badly.

First I phoned my mum. She was staying with a friend in a caravan and the signal was really bad.

When she answered the phone her silence told me she already knew something. 'Mum,' I sobbed. 'Mum, I've got cancer. Mum?'

But all I got was . . . nothing. Total silence. She couldn't speak. She quite often gets like this in difficult situations—she just freezes up—but now wasn't the time for it.

'Mum,' I shouted. 'Stop it! Stop! I need you. I need you more than ever. Come on, be a mum.'

I grew more and more angry as she carried on saying nothing. Not a word.

'You've never been a mother to me!' I screamed and slammed the phone down.

I was so angry. Why couldn't she just put me first for once? It wasn't about her—it was about me. I needed her to be strong for me, but she couldn't do it, not then.

It had always just been Mum and me so I understood why this news would shatter her world. She split with my druggie dad when I was about a year old. She found a gun under my cot that she knew must have been his. She kicked him out straight away and he ended up in and out of prison until he died when I was twenty-three. So it's only ever been the two of us, but our relationship has had its ups and downs over the years, as anyone who has read my autobiography will know! Let's just say that a lot of the time I've had to be the mother rather than her.

I came off the phone seething that she couldn't find some words to comfort me at a time like this. But it was devastating news for her as well and I didn't want us to fall out.

Fifteen minutes later I rang back. 'I'm so sorry,' I said. 'I am really sorry.'

'So am I, Jade,' she sobbed. 'Ring me when you get home.'

I lay down and cried, feeling so alone.

Next I rang Danielle, a good mate of mine for the last seven years. We're both single mums and often hang out together. She was on holiday in Portugal.

'I've got cancer,' I said as soon as she answered the phone.

'Oh, Jade!' she cried, really upset. 'I can't believe it! What have they said to you? How serious is it?'

I'd thought I wasn't really hearing the doctor's words in the Diary Room in my shocked state, but something he'd said came back to me. 'They say it's grade two, whatever that means.'

Danielle was really sweet but the fact that she sounded so upset was upsetting me as well. I hung up, promising to call her as soon as I got home.

Next I called Jack, my on-again–off-again

boyfriend of the last three years. Mark had already told him, so at least he didn't find out from the TV or something.

'You're going to be okay,' he said. But how did anyone know that?

'I've got cancer,' I kept repeating over and over. I think I was just trying to get my head around it.

'Doctors can do all sorts of things these days,' said Jack. 'They've caught it early on. You can deal with this. I'll be there for you every step of the way.'

We talked for a few hours and he really helped to calm me down. After we came off the phone I managed to get a bit of sleep, which by that stage I really needed. But when I wakened in the early hours of the morning, it was the first thought in my head: 'I've got cancer.'

19th August 2008

I got on the Virgin flight home to Heathrow just feeling numb. The *Big Brother* producers sent someone from the team with me, but I didn't know him so I had no one to talk to in the airport or on the flight.

Usually when I sit down on a plane I'm excited to see what films are showing and what's going to be on the menu. I love those little tiny portions of airline food set out on a tray, with the packets of salt and pepper and the freshening wipe. Now I had no interest in anything.

I didn't want to smile or chat to anyone because all I could think of was that C-word.

I have cancer.

I wanted to get home and for my mum to rub my head the way she sometimes did and tell me everything would be okay.

I tried to close my eyes and think of my boys. Most of all I longed to touch their soft skin and kiss their cheeks so hard. I wanted to hold them like I'd never done before.

I tried to just listen to the hum of the plane engines and ignore the sound of babies crying and moody passengers asking for more drinks or extra blankets.

I didn't want anything now except my family.

I pushed a pillow up against the window, closed my eyes and thought of Jack.

Imagining him holding me and telling me it was all a dream made me feel a bit better.

As all these thoughts were rushing through my mind, I wanted to scream 'Why me?'

Just when I was getting on with my life and putting all the bad things behind me. My mum becoming a crack addict when I was eighteen; my dad's horrible death of a heroin overdose in a Kentucky Fried Chicken restaurant; my bad relationships; the racism row over my argument with Shilpa Shetty. Why is the Big Man in the Sky giving me another challenge?

Then I suddenly got this really weird feeling.

I don't know how to explain it but I thought that if my life was in danger, it was about time I sorted it all out. It made me want to do special things.

Like make peace with my dad. He's dead, so why do I still hate him? I decided I would go and put some flowers on his grave.

I wanted to see my half-brothers: my dad's son Miles, who I'd never even met before, and my

9

mum's son Brett.

I wanted truly, properly to forgive my mum. To tell her none of the past mattered any more.

Bobby and Freddy were only five and three but I decided I wanted to take my two special boys to a poor country and let them see that what they have—all the toys and holidays and the nice home—is not like that for everyone. I wanted them to appreciate the things we had.

And, for me this is weird, I wanted to reach out somehow and find a religion.

I never listened in my RE lessons at school—or any lessons at school for that matter—and I don't know much about God and religious stuff. Churches always seemed like a place for other people.

Now I was forced to think about dying I wanted to understand about living. For I could suddenly see that despite everything I've had—like my kids, houses, money and fame—I hadn't really deeply appreciated it, because I didn't think I had to.

I didn't want to feel any more anger. I wanted to be at peace with everyone now.

I sat and thought about the list of things I wanted to do as the plane carried me back home to my family thousands of miles away. I had no idea how long I might have to do them all so I'd have to get started straight away. Just in case.

20th August 2008

The flight took eleven hours and it was the following morning when we landed at Heathrow. I unclipped my seatbelt and felt myself welling up

10

again.

For the past nine years, since *Big Brother 3* in 2002, I have lived my life in the spotlight and I knew this would be no different. I'll never forget that moment when I stepped outside the *Big Brother* house and saw those cameras flashing and realised: 'Oh my god, I must be famous!'

But landing at Heathrow that morning I wished I could switch it all off for the day.

An air stewardess led me to the VIP lounge. I put my arm through hers and walked as fast as I could. My legs still felt like jelly. I wanted to run away and hide.

The word 'cancer' seemed to be etched behind my eyes and echoing round my head.

Then I spotted a big horde of photographers waiting for me.

I could hear the clicking of the camera shutters as I approached. I kept my head down but my feet were lighting up with flashes as I stumbled across the swirly-patterned carpet.

I'm used to being in the spotlight, and usually a few paps don't bother me at all. This time, though, I felt the heat of the lights and all those eyes on me and I felt so vulnerable, as if I'd forgotten to put my clothes on.

I clenched my lips together and my heart started to beat really fast. I didn't want to cry again, but the tears were never far from the surface.

Then there was another huge flash and the tears began dripping from my eyelashes. Of course that made them snap away even more. That's what they wanted: Tragic Jade Breaks Down; Jade In Tears at Cancer Diagnosis.

We got outside with the help of a police escort

and I threw myself onto the back seat of the car. I felt safer away from the spotlight.

I switched my phone on and straight away lots of texts came through. Carly, my friend who helped me open my Ugly beauty salon, had sent me a text saying she'd heard the news and was thinking of me. I was glad she'd got in touch. We'd drifted apart a bit after the salon closed but now I wanted to make peace with everyone. Having cancer makes you realise any bad feelings are just not worth it.

Of course, if she had heard that meant it had been reported in the press already. It figured. When you get your diagnosis on TV, you're not going to keep it secret for long because even though the producers edited it out, it would have appeared on the internet.

I watched the motorway rushing past the window.

'You know, Jade,' I thought, *'it isn't that bad. It can't be. You're a mum. You need to be here and live for your boys. You can't possibly die; you're just too young. You've got cancer; you'll get it sorted.'*

Why would this happen to me anyway? I'd taken more crap than most people, so why this as well? On top of everything else, why cancer?

Come on, Jade. Worse things have happened. Surely. Haven't they?

Images of bald people crowded my head. Very sick people with oxygen tanks by their beds and tubes in their arms. Hospitals. Treatments.

Fuck it, it IS bad. It's cancer! You don't get much more serious than that . . .

By the time I'd reached my house, I felt a bit calmer. Almost convinced this couldn't be real.

I spotted the shadows of photographers outside my house and kept my head down as I opened the door.

They shouted at me: 'Jade, Jade, are you okay? How do you feel?'

Well, how did they think I felt?

Normally, you just try and stop me from saying something. I open my mouth and say whatever jumps into my head. All too often the words bypass my brain so I end up getting into trouble again. But this time was different. My whole world had changed.

That old Jade had gone and now the words were stuck in my throat. My mouth felt so dry, I wanted to get myself inside the house and away from all the media.

I rang the bell and waited for Jack to answer. I was so relieved when the door opened and I saw him holding out his arms that I just walked right into them. I felt small and weak and helpless as he squeezed me tightly. Funny, because we weren't even supposed to be officially together at that time—whatever 'officially' means.

We'd split up ten months earlier because we were always rowing and having ups and downs. He was six years younger than me and could be a bit immature. He certainly wasn't ready for the media spotlight that came with being my boyfriend. Paps were always catching him out with his arm round girls in clubs or whatever, and sometimes I knew it was an innocent thing, but not always. But despite everything, I knew I had a friend in Jack, so we'd always carried on seeing each other and spending time with each other. We couldn't seem to keep away.

13

And there is no one who gives me hugs like he does. You know the ones where your problems all seem to melt away?

'Jack,' I cried. 'I'm so scared.'

He just hugged me and kept repeating that it was going to be okay.

He'd been staying in my house as he'd promised me he'd decorate the rooms while I was away in India. As I glanced around I could see that obviously he hadn't had time to get very far, but I certainly wasn't going to say anything about it that day.

I hadn't even wanted to go to India at first, because Jack was due to go to court for bashing someone with a golf club the previous December and I was afraid he'd be in prison when I got back.

I had no doubt that he really cared about me but he kept screwing up and things had been difficult between us. He had a great relationship with my boys, though, and that meant a lot. And he was there for me when I really needed him— like today.

Freddy and Bobby had been staying with Jeff, their father, while I was in India and were due to come back to me in a few days' time. I really wanted to see them straight away but had hospital trips already arranged for the next few days so I wouldn't have been able to look after them anyway. Jeff is a good dad—I had no worries there. It was just selfish of me to want to see them for comfort, for the special little hugs that only three-year-olds and five-year-olds can give you. But maybe it was best that they didn't see me in such a state.

I called Mum but she said it would be a few days

more before she could get back. I got the impression she didn't really understand the seriousness of the situation but there was nothing more I could say until I'd seen the doctors. I've had loads of scares in the past so she probably thought it was just another one, but I knew this was something more. No one had actually told me I had cancer before.

I was so tired after all the crying, I didn't feel hungry. My head was all over the place from the different time zones. India is about five hours ahead of England, I think—or is it the other way round? Anyway, we went to bed early. Usually I feel totally relaxed in my warm, soft giant bed. I love my bedroom with its high ceiling and massive TV. It's always been my special place.

This time, everything felt different. Soon my pillow was soaked with tears, and I lay there in a panic with my heart thudding. Not to feel all safe and snuggly in your own bed is horrible.

Jack wrapped his arms around me, speaking softly in my ear.

'You'll be okay. I'm here,' he whispered. 'I'm here every step of the way.'

Although his words couldn't take the horrible cancer away, they made me soften inside.

We talked and I sobbed for ages until sleep overcame me and the room finally went dark.

Chapter Two

Lots of Tests

21st August 2008

As soon as I woke up and remembered what was happening, I felt sick. There was an appointment booked for me that morning at Harlow Hospital— the one where doctors had told me over and over again I was okay.

I got ready to go, my legs like jelly. Jack was coming too, thank God.

My hands were so sweaty it was as though I'd just washed them. They were shaking as well, like I was an old drunk or something.

The doctors examined me again then told me they wanted me to do an MRI scan.

I spoke to Mark while we waited. He told me the papers had already brought out the stories of me having cancer and he read out a few of the headlines. I'm used to seeing my name in headlines but not next to the word 'cancer'. That kept bringing it home to me again and again. 'Jade Goody has cancer'. If they said it, it must be true— or not, because we all know they're not always right, don't we?

After a while we were led to a room with a big, scary-looking machine I'd never seen before. I had to lie down on it and was told to keep still as it started making loads of noise. All that was going through my head was: *'Oh my god, this is real.'*

I was beginning to wonder if I could trust any

doctors at all when all the time they'd been saying I was okay when I actually had cancer. As the machine went whirring round, I thought: '*This was supposed to be just bad periods. What on earth am I doing here?*'

It felt as though I was being buried alive in there. There was a plastic mask that came right down close to my face and I had to lie very still. I'm such a fidget, that was really hard to do. And I was all on my own inside that machine. No one could hold my hand or whisper nice things to me. I wouldn't have been able to hear over the noise.

I just started thinking about stuff. *Cancer is so serious . . . This is happening to me . . . Why me? . . . I'm glad it was Jack that came with me . . . I'm scared of what they are going to find.*

It was pretty weird but it seemed that Jack and I were a couple again. We'd been through good times and bad. Very bad. But it said a lot that he was the one I wanted by my side when I had a scan for cancer. That's when you know who really matters in your life.

After the scan, a woman doctor told me it looked as though just the neck of the womb was affected. I know it sounds silly but it always makes me feel weird when they talk about a 'neck' down there. Where's the head then?

The doctor said: 'We can just cut it away and you may need some radiotherapy and chemo.'

I thought to myself: 'Oh crap.' I knew that chemotherapy was the one that made you lose your hair and throw up a lot, and radiotherapy sounded like radiation from a nuclear accident, the kind that makes you have three-headed babies.

Then she told me there was still hope so it

17

wasn't that bad.

I was just confused about all the different messages I was getting. The main thing I wanted people to answer me was: 'Was I going to be okay?' *Please, God, yes.* But no one was saying one way or the other.

*   *   *

As soon as we left Harlow Hospital we had to head up to London. Max Clifford, who has been my publicist for some time now, was well concerned about the whole thing and had made me an appointment with a private Harley Street doctor, Dr Ann Coxon. He said he'd pay for a private scan. I couldn't speak, I was so grateful. What a good man he was for doing that! If he'd been there I'd have hugged him.

One of my good friends Charlene met Jack and me for the appointment. I've known Charlene for years, since we grew up near each other in Bermondsey. We made our way to the swanky Harley Street address I'd been told and were shown in to the doctor's office, where Dr Coxon explained what was going to happen.

She wanted me to have another scan but this would be different from the Harlow one because I had to have an injection beforehand and she told me I had to breathe in and out several times. This scan would show loads of new angles and bits of my body I never knew I had! It was much more detailed than the one in Harlow. Jack wasn't allowed in this time. He and Charlene sat outside in the posh waiting room looking through the magazines.

Because I'd just had a scan done the day before, I didn't feel so scared—just a bit confused because it was different to the last one. I followed all the instructions and while I was inside the scanner I tried to think about nice things to take my mind off it all. I thought about the boys when they were babies, and all the cute things they had said and done when they were toddlers, and I thought about how much I was looking forward to seeing them in a couple of days' time.

At last it was over, but Dr Coxon said I'd have to come back the next day for the results, so Jack and I piled into the car and went home.

*   *   *

I'm not much of a reader usually, but a couple of people had hinted to me that there were some horrible things written about me on the internet. That evening I went to look them up and was really upset at what I found:

'Can't believe Jade Goody is talking about having cancer when it's just a few abnormal cells. Loads of people get that.'

'I have no sympathy with Jade Goody. It's like karma. She said all those horrible racist things to Shilpa Shetty and then she got cancer . . .'

'Jade is exaggerating and lying about this cancer and I think she should be ashamed . . .'

What kind of sicko would make up a story that they had cancer? That's something I'd never dream of doing. Some people are sick in the head. I've read some rubbish written about me over the years but this took the biscuit.

Call me a racist, a bigot, a chav, whatever—but

don't call me a liar, especially not over this.

I've said sorry so many times over the Shilpa Shetty incident. And I really mean it. I wish I could go back and do things differently but I can't, and that's that.

Just thinking about me on that film makes me feel ill. But how could people say I deserve this killer disease because of some mistakes I made two years ago? That really is a nasty thing to say to anyone.

Some internet bloggers were asking why I had suddenly had a medical test just before I headed off to India if I didn't want to make some publicity thing out of it. Well, I'd been having those tests for years and years. I'd had my first smear aged sixteen, after which I had laser treatment to remove abnormal cells. Then a second one at eighteen and more laser treatment. At twenty-two I was pregnant with Bobby, then I had Freddy and after that my smears were normal. I had a miscarriage with Jack's baby in June 2007 and had an abnormal smear then but doctors didn't seem worried about it. Test after test said there was no cancer.

Nothing seemed to need doing.

Within months after the miscarriage I was admitted to hospital with agonising pains. They gave me an ultrasound and said that was normal.

The horrible pain and awful heavy bleeding kept coming back over the next few months and I kept going back trying to find answers but I was hitting a brick wall.

One doctor even said to me: 'You're an attention-seeking hysteric and wouldn't know a normal period even if it hit you.'

I felt awful. They thought I was making things up. I didn't think I was a hypo-whatever-it's-called, but if a doctor tells you you are then you believe him. Maybe these were just normal periods I was having? Maybe I had a low pain threshold? How could I be ill when every medical person I saw said I wasn't?

So I just took the hospital doctors' decisions on faith. I'd had lots of tests and then I had another dose of laser treatment in August 2007 but they'd said it was fine for me to go to India.

If I'd known the news, I'd never have gone. As a mum, my health is too important. I hope all those people who doubted me are ashamed of themselves.

It was one of the tests I'd had on that last visit that came out positive. No one else had picked this up.

Reading the internet stuff that night was devastating. Obviously there were lots of members of the public who still hated me over the Shilpa thing. It was horrible and upsetting on top of all the rest of the bad news I was getting.

I just curled up in a ball. I wanted to shut out the world. I didn't answer the phone, and when Jack asked me what I wanted for dinner I said I wasn't hungry. I had such a huge lump in my throat I couldn't have swallowed a single thing.

22nd August 2008

Jack came with me the next day to get the results of the scan, and I was really glad he had because it was devastating.

When I got to the Royal Marsden Hospital, the famous cancer hospital in London, I had a meeting with a surgeon called Dr Tom Ind. He seemed like a straight kind of man. I'm getting used to meeting all these posh doctors now.

He said to me: 'I work one on one with my patients. I give them all the information and tell them the truth upfront about what's going on. If you don't want this, I can refer you to someone else who works differently.'

I decided there and then that he was the best of the best and I wanted to go with him. There was no point in people trying to be tactful and not telling it to me like it was.

He said he had already been studying my case. I can't believe I'm being called 'a case'. It makes me feel as if my body is something separate from me.

He said that more cancer had shown up and I had a great big tumour that filled half my womb. He wanted to do a mini operation that takes about fifteen minutes to remove some of the tissue and see exactly what this cancer is doing.

I knew he was giving it to me like it was. I was terrified, of course, but also relieved in a weird way because at last someone seemed to know what they were talking about.

'What does it mean?' I asked.

Then he told me some news I wasn't expecting. He said once they were inside and had a look, there was a 50–50 chance I'd need a radical . . . whatever it's called where they take out your womb (a hysterectomy, someone just told me).

I don't know much about biological things, but even I knew that meant no more kids.

'Oh my god,' I cried. 'You're joking!'

A sick pain hurt my heart right inside. *No more babies. Ever.*

My chin wobbled as I looked at Jack and realised what that meant for him. We couldn't have kids together. And I'd always wished for a little girl. I'd always thought I'd have a daughter one day. Now she'll never be born.

Thank God I've got my boys.

Then he started telling me all the percentages of whether I was going to live or die, and obviously that was horrible. It didn't feel real. It was as though he was talking about someone else.

He told me first of all that if the cancer had spread there was a 55 per cent chance I could die. But if it hadn't, there was a 95 per cent chance I would live. I was never any good at maths but 95 sounded a lot better than 55.

He said that if the cancer had spread to my bloodstream my major organs, like the liver and kidneys, were at risk.

They wouldn't be able to tell me till after I'd had the operation though.

I was bloody terrified.

He explained that after the op, I would have to have radiotherapy and chemotherapy.

My mouth fell open like a goldfish. 'Excuse me?' I asked.

I got him to repeat stuff and gradually it started to sink in. I might need my whole womb out and really strong treatment afterwards. Radiotherapy to burn the cells and chemo to kill the cancer.

The only good news was that he said they could try to save my ovaries, so I could maybe have kids still.

'What would have happened if I'd stayed in

23

Indian *Big Brother*?' I asked.

Without hesitation he said: 'Jade, you would have ended up with incurable cancer within three months.'

I felt my insides go all funny. 'Oh my god!' I said. 'Oh my god!' Jack just squeezed my hand and stared at the floor.

Being told you could have been months from death is the scariest thing in the world. I suppose we can all be moments away from death without knowing it—like if you accidentally step out in front of a car or something—but to know that it could have been happening to you in a few months . . . I felt really wobbly.

Putting on a brave face is something I am used to doing. I could see in Jack's eyes how scared he was for me, so I tried to crack a joke. I can't remember what. I'm sure it wasn't very funny.

All of a sudden, I realised I was at the beginning of a long, long journey full of tests and hospitals and treatments. This wasn't going to be over quickly.

*   *   *

What would I tell the boys? Instinctively, I wanted to hide it from them, protect them. They are too young to know about horrible things like cancer.

Thinking of the boys, deep in my heart I made a big decision. I was going to fight this damn thing every step of the way. I wouldn't let it win. Whatever I had to do, no matter how painful or horrible, then I would do it. I would take any drugs they wanted me to take and have any operations I needed to have because I had to beat this cancer.

There was no other option.

I had to get through it because I had Bobby and Freddy to live for. And that was the bottom line.

*   *   *

After getting the scan results I had to go to the Soho Hotel to have an interview with a journalist from the *Sun* about my cancer. I was going to put my side of it and try to answer some of the people who had been saying I was doing it as a publicity stunt. Of course, people might ask why I was bothering to give a press interview when I was so ill. But it's always been my way of coping. *Just put a smile on your face and carry on, Jade.*

Katherine Lister did the interview. She used to work alongside my old agent John Noel years ago and I knew and trusted her.

Mark was there throughout and Jack lay on a bed texting his mates and occasionally reaching over to squeeze my hand. He'd hardly said a word since we heard the news from Dr Ind and I think he was in shock. We both were.

As I talked to Katherine about my illness I kept turning to Mark and Jack and saying: 'I can't believe this.' I really couldn't.

Shit, I really do have cancer. It felt more real now I was telling someone else but just saying the words 'I've got cancer' was incredibly hard. Inside I still felt as though I was talking about someone else.

Then—oh my god—I started bawling when they took the pictures. That's just me though; I cry so easily anyway.

I knew I was going to look terrible.

25

I've lived my life through the press but it's a bit different when it's something so serious. I do deal with things better when they are out there, but never ever ever did I imagine I'd be told I had cancer on a reality TV show. I mean, how fucked up is that?

*   *   *

After the interview and the photos were all done, Mark, Jack and I went downstairs for a snack. We sat on this lovely cream sofa in the library area of the hotel, chatting away. It was nice to see Mark and I was starting to feel almost like my normal self when a terrible cramping pain made me double up.

Jack and Mark carried on talking, not realising anything was wrong, but I could feel a wetness on my bum and looked down to see a red oozing patch.

I wanted the ground to open up and swallow me! How embarrassing is that? Bleeding in a posh hotel on a cream sofa.

I got up and hobbled over to the reception. Thank God the manager was a lady.

I was bent over, looking like a nutter, and I said: 'I'm so sorry I'm not well. I've just bled all over your nice sofa. Is there anywhere I can clean myself up?'

She looked surprised, then said: 'Please don't worry.' She led me to a toilet to clean up and she found me a nice white dressing gown to put on over my stained clothes. She couldn't have been more sweet about it.

I washed myself and put the dressing gown on,

26

while she went off to tell the guys what had happened. Mark called a cab to pick us up at the side entrance of the hotel and I slipped out. Thank God no one was waiting. I just wanted to escape home again.

There was no holding back in the car. I cried my eyes out. Jack rubbed my back as I sobbed, feeling like an old lady.

'It's okay, babe, it's okay,' he said.

'I'm so embarrassed, Jack,' I sobbed. 'It's not fair. I just want it all to go away.'

He held me for a bit then passed me my mobile.

'Call the boys, babe. They'll cheer you up.'

So I did, and you know what? He was right. He knows me so well. It was just so lovely to hear their little voices telling me about all the things they'd been doing, and saying they missed me. 'I miss you too,' I said, half smiling and half on the point of tears again.

*   *   *

That evening Jack and I went to the cinema with my friend Jen. We started playing a game in the car where we took turns to sing along to songs on the radio and CDs. When one person stopped, the next person had to make up funny words to finish the song and we ended up cracking up with laughter. It felt so good to do something normal and not think about cancer.

At one point Jen said: 'You two are so sweet together.'

It's true, we have a good laugh. He can make me giggle more than just about anyone else I've ever met. In a way we get on because I act younger than

27

I am and he acts older (well, sometimes he does—not always!).

Back home again, I talked to Jack about the news. My body, the one that was making all this cancer, didn't feel like my own any more. It probably wouldn't be able to make more babies and that meant I didn't feel like the woman I once was.

I got into bed for a cuddle, really tired out. My mind was racing away, thinking about the baby I'd wanted to have with Jack one day and the way that had been taken away from us.

I'd already had a miscarriage with his baby, and now this.

It was losing something we never had, but it was still really painful. I had kids myself, but if Jack and I stayed together was it fair to ask him to give up the chance of ever having a baby himself?

My thoughts were whirring on and on. I wanted to sleep but couldn't.

All I wanted was Jack and my boys. I couldn't wait for Bobby and Freddy to get back from Jeff's. I was just counting the minutes until I could see them and wrap them up in my arms.

23rd August 2008

My interview in the *Sun* came out today so I picked up a copy on the way to the Royal Marsden. The photos were every bit as bad as I thought. I look terrible and felt so sad when I saw them. I wish people would stop taking my picture when I've been crying my eyes out. I've lived my life in the public eye since I came out of the Big Brother

28

house in 2002 but it's a bit different when it's something so serious.

I'm going to have the mini operation today to see what's going on. Inside I feel totally numb. I have to try and help them get to the bottom of this. I have to focus on getting well.

*   *   *

I woke up after the operation, feeling really groggy. Dr Ind came to tell me the results. He said they had found a tiny bit of cancer that had escaped into the outside bit of my womb, which is not great news. This makes the percentage survival rate much less. It means it has spread and I will definitely need the whole womb taken out, followed by chemo and radio. He said there's no chance I can have another baby now.

I took the news really calmly again. Inside I felt cut up about losing that last little window of hope but I'd already known it was unlikely I'd be able to have more babies.

He carried on, telling me that I've been referred to Dr Peter Blake and Professor Martin Gore, who are part of the oncology team at the Royal Marsden. I am going to have an initial treatment of radiotherapy and chemotherapy to start with and then stronger chemo later after my operation.

The radiotherapy will be every day and the chemo once a week on Thursdays.

Charlene and Jack came in to sit with me as I recovered from the operation. She said she'd come with me for the chemo and radiotherapy too.

'No, don't,' I said. 'I'll probably fall asleep during the treatments and you'll only be bored.'

'I really don't mind, Jade,' she said.

'No, no, don't,' I replied. I didn't want to put anyone out. I've always looked after myself and everyone else around me as well and that's what I'm going to carry on doing now.

24th August 2008

Back at home the morning after, my eyes were all gritty because of lack of sleep. I don't feel as though I will ever be able to just curl up and drop off naturally again. Every time I close my eyes, all the horrible things about the cancer start spinning around in my head.

The worst bit is finally dropping off then waking up again and knowing nothing has changed. I am still me and the cancer is still there, growing inside me.

I turned over and felt a squishy damp patch.

'Urgh!' I yelled, touching it with my hands.

The sheets were soaked in blood. I felt so disgusting and embarrassed.

I got up, washed myself off and stripped the sheets for washing. It wasn't my fault. I shouldn't beat myself up about it. I tried to put it to the back of my mind. Really, it was the least of my worries.

My next instinct was to ring the people I cared about and tell them, just to get it off my chest.

One of the first people I rang was my friend Kate Jackson, who was filming in Afghanistan. She's a producer for Granada TV and I met her when I was filming one of my TV shows, *Jade's Salon*, in 2005.

'Kate, I've got cancer. I can't believe it,' I

sobbed down the line to her mobile, thousands of miles away. 'What am I gonna do?'

Kate took a deep breath. 'We'll do what we always do. The Fab Four will get together and we will fight this. You are going to be okay, Jade.'

The Fab Four are: me, Kate, Simon Bridger and Danny Hayward. The boys are photographers I met after I got out of *Big Brother 3* and they are living proof that press photographers can be really nice guys, even if that's not the way lots of people see them.

The Fab Four get together for dinner parties about once a month and put the world to rights. They're such good mates. I can trust them with my life, something that can be hard to do in this game.

I carried on crying but Kate's words did make me feel a bit better.

It's good to know I have them on my side in this stupid, crazy fight against the Big C. I'm going to need my friends Big Time.

Chapter Three

Getting Away From It All

25th August 2008

The boys are back! I just rushed to the door and swept them up in my arms. They seemed really pleased to see me, and Jack as well. I had to be careful not to crush them I wanted to hold them so tightly. It made me feel more sane having them with me again because I have a routine and things to do to look after them: meals, playing, bathing and so on.

I've booked us all a holiday in Carmarthenshire in West Wales—me, Jack and the boys. It'll be a chance to spend some proper family time together.

'We're gonna go to a beach, go fishing, horse-riding, everything!' I told them.

Danny and Simon said they would drive down there with us so they can take some snaps. I hope they know the way because I haven't a clue!

27th August 2008

We're off on our family holiday. Hopefully there won't be so much drama as on the last big family holiday to Tobago, when a bush fire almost reached our villa and I was out in the road hurling buckets of water at it!

We're staying in a converted stable next to a

guesthouse. It took us ages to get here. It's so remote that the sat navs weren't working, which is a disaster for me! I've never understood maps. I've never figured out what happens when the line runs out at the end of the page. I mean, where does it go next?

Anyway, we arrived really late and put the boys straight to bed.

It's beautiful up here and so good to have fresh air on our faces. It's also good to have a chance to spend some time doing different things. I want a proper rural English holiday. (Someone just told me that Wales is not in England. Is that true?)

No jet skis and diamonds for me. Fresh air and green fields is what I need just now.

28th August 2008

We're going fishing today! I'm feeling all countrified and excited about it. The horrible hospitals seem a million miles away.

The four of us laughed all day long, stomping in the mud in our wellies, even though Jack and I hate wearing those rubbery things. They look so silly and feel cold on our feet but it's better that than getting wet, muddy socks.

We couldn't wait to get down to the river and we hired rods from the local angling people. They gave us a bucket of wriggling worms as well. Poor Bobby didn't want to touch the wrigglers. He was freaking out a bit, wrinkling his nose and shouting if I put one near him. Meanwhile Freddy was trying to put them in his pockets, which was making me wet myself laughing.

I love watching my boys playing together. They are such different personalities. Bobby is quite sensitive—he can tell when things aren't right—and he's very loving. Freddy is a gorgeous kid too but is much more wild. He never stops tearing around and can be quite mischievous.

To tell you the truth, I wasn't any good at fishing—none of us were. We were all crap and gave up before long as we weren't catching anything. It's boring just sitting on a riverbank waiting. I've never been very good at waiting!

Afterwards we went horse-riding. The boys were going crazy over the horses, they loved them so much. They were both asking: 'Please can we get one?' What with the dogs and my boys to look after, I said that horses were the last thing we needed right now.

They all had a good go on them, including Jack. I did too.

I used to love horse-riding when I was younger. My dad had a rich girlfriend at one point and she let me use their horses. It was amazing.

Jack was a bit nervous though. He made me laugh, pulling faces and wanting to get off. He didn't like the horse moving and said it hurt his bits.

I wasn't letting him give up that easily, though. 'Let's go for a trot,' I suggested.

I could tell he wanted to keep up with me because he knew he'd never hear the last of it otherwise! I couldn't stop laughing as he tried to cling onto the reins.

'What is trotting anyway?' he shouted.

Ha, ha! The boys were braver than him!

When he jumped down he couldn't walk

properly and was staggering around like John Wayne. It cracked me up.

For a whole five minutes, all the laughing made me forget I am ill.

Then I went to the toilet and remembered all over again because thick, black, tarry stuff was falling out of me into the loo. It smelled disgusting and made me feel horrible inside.

*　　　*　　　*

It's like a mad rollercoaster—one minute I'm laughing with my boys and can forget about cancer and the next it hits me hard again.

The pain was bad, like really severe period pains.

I called Dr Ind on my mobile and he explained that it was the cancer causing bits of my womb to come away.

People use the expression 'I'm falling apart'. Well, right now I really am.

*　　　*　　　*

Later on I got the Scrabble board out. Before you laugh, we are actually not that bad. I can spell enough words to play with my two clever little boys. They may be at a better school than I ever went to, but if I can't spell as well as a three-year-old and a five-year-old I'm really in trouble.

I felt so tired when the sun went down that I went to bed early, still feeling the cramps.

It all catches up on me once the boys are asleep.

29th August 2008

Not a nice day. It started out badly and just got worse. Jack woke up with the hump but wouldn't tell me why. I still had horrible tummy pains and the boys were fighting with each other.

I always put on my biggest smile when things are this bad. I took some painkillers, made the breakfast and thought: 'Keep smiling, Mum! Just keep smiling.'

We all went on a boat trip out to sea and Bobby totally loved it. The water was calming and everyone was happy again.

We went to see porpooses (or whatever that name is for animals like dolphins and seals). I didn't know you could get seals in England.

The trip lasted a couple of hours but when we got back to shore Bobby wanted to go straight back out again.

'No, Bobby,' I said. 'We are going for some food now. We're hungry.'

He screwed his face up into a ball and screamed like you wouldn't believe. 'I want another go!' he yelled. 'It's not fair!'

I know where he gets his lungs from, I suppose. Can't duck out of that one.

I dragged him away while all the other tourists were staring and obviously thinking he was a spoilt brat.

'I want to hear "thank you, Mum" not screaming, Bobby,' I snapped at him. 'You're being really ungrateful after I've given you a nice treat.'

I managed to get him into the car and strapped him in, but the noise of his crying upset me so much that I began to cry. Soon I was sobbing my head off. I hated myself for telling him off. He's only little and doesn't have any idea what's going on with me. I hate seeing my boys upset.

Jack was at a loss to know what to do.

I told Bobby to say sorry and, bless his heart, he started crying and gave me a hug.

'I'm sorry, Mummy,' he sobbed.

'I'm sorry for shouting at you,' I cried, then we had the biggest cuddle.

Every time we have a cuddle now, I feel myself well up. It's so hard when I think about the future and what might happen. *But I won't let myself think that way. I can't.*

*   *   *

That night my emotions were all over the place. I told Jack that I couldn't be with him any more because I could never give him a family of his own.

'It's not fair that I put you through this,' I said. 'It's going to be so hard.'

I meant it too. He's still only young, a twenty-one-year-old boy. We've been through so much together—breaking up, making up, even cheating death in a car accident in 2007. Oh, and that was before we were kidnapped by a mad taxi driver who picked us up in London a few months earlier. And, of course, my miscarriage. But fighting cancer and not being able to have kids was too much.

Looking back, it makes the miscarriage even more painful. Jack couldn't wait to be a dad. I think his mum was a bit worried as he was only nineteen at the time—I'd have been worried if that was Bobby or Freddy—but she soon came round.

37

My mum went out and bought loads of baby clothes. She thought it was going to be a girl. *The girl I will never have.*

I did an interview in *OK!* about it and even had some photos taken of my three months' bump. We were really looking forward to having a baby of our own. Now I can never ever give him that.

He keeps trying to make a joke out of it, saying: 'I've already got two kids—that's quite enough, thanks!'

I can't laugh about it. 'You might want a family of your own one day and I don't want to deny you that,' I said. 'You should just leave me and get on with it, Jack.'

He looked at me in the eye and shook his head. 'I already have a family,' he said. 'You, me, Bobby and Freddy. I'm not going anywhere.'

'But I'm not going to be like a real woman any more,' I cried. 'What's the point in us having a relationship?'

I felt so low, so sad inside.

He kissed me over and over, telling me I was a great mum. 'And you'll make a great wife too,' he said, lifting up my chin. 'With or without hair.'

I was all snotty but couldn't help giggling. He was joking, I think, but little did he know I'd been thinking a lot about the two of us since my cancer was discovered, and the idea was forming in my head that I really wanted to marry Jack. He was such a good father figure to my boys, and no matter how many dramas he and I went through we always seemed to get back together in the end.

But he was just a twenty-one-year-old. Boys that age don't want to get married. I shouldn't get my hopes up just because I was ill. I tried to put the thought out of my head, but in bed that night after he fell asleep I was looking at him and thinking to myself: 'Mr and Mrs Tweed. Who knows?'

30th August 2008

We found a lovely beach near our guesthouse. It was sandy with a big cliff and no one was there. It was like our own private beach. We just set up some deckchairs and let the boys start playing in the sea and sand and they loved it. It wasn't even a hot day. It was a bit cloudy but that didn't matter.

'I love it here,' I said to Jack. 'I really want to buy a house here and when I am better we can come here all the time. It's good for the boys.'

I like watching Jack play with them. He's like a big kid himself sometimes and they idolise him.

This evening I started to cry again. I can't help it. I hide my feelings all day for the kids but they have to come out some time, usually after they've gone to bed. Jack just cuddled me and kept saying everything would be okay. I'll try and believe him. He's been brilliant through all of this—sweet and kind and saying all the right things. I wish everyone could see this wonderful side of him instead of the image they all have of him out on the town getting drunk and making trouble.

Chapter Four

Losing Jack

31st August 2008

We had to come back today because Jack is due in court tomorrow. I'm praying he doesn't get sent to prison. Deep down I think he will get off. I've been trying not to think about it because I can't face the thought of losing him and he doesn't seem to want to talk about it either. He says he doesn't want me in court with him and I'll respect that.

I know he was wrong to bash that man over the head with a golf club. Like I've said before, Jack can be a real Jekyll and Hyde character after he's had a drink. But at the end of the day he is really, truly sorry, and in my mind that's what counts. He admits he did wrong and, hopefully, has learned his lesson. People seem to forget he's only twenty-one and at that age men make their mistakes.

We watched a DVD and had a takeaway and I tried to blank it out. We'll just have to hope for the best.

In many ways I feel so protective towards Jack. He gets loads of flak whatever he does. No one seems to realise just how lovely he can be to me, and especially to my boys. They adore him.

I'll never forget when I went on the Jonathan Ross show and he made a point of talking to me in the dressing room afterwards, telling me that Jack is a wrong 'un for me.

40

I was touched he cared that much about me—he is a dad himself after all—but I wanted to tell him Jack's not all bad. He just gets slated in the press all the time no matter whether he deserves it or not.

I'm having more than my fair share of bad luck at the moment so I hope that to balance things up Jack can have some good luck in court tomorrow. Fingers, toes and everything else is crossed for him.

1st September 2008

I went on *GMTV* today to talk about the cancer. I wanted to set the record straight about a few things.

Like the fact that I certainly didn't know I had cancer when I went in the Indian *Big Brother* house, because the doctors had told me my bleeding was just stress or bad periods. And that I'd already signed up to do the Living TV show *Living with Jade* long before any of this cancer nightmare started and it had nothing to do with it.

I never really plan what I'm going to say—it just all sort of comes out.

I told Fiona Phillips that I am not made of iron. I know people think I am strong, which is lovely, but this is tough.

I think maybe the first shock is wearing off because I'm not crying all the time any more and I managed not to cry too much on TV.

But after the show, I had two bits of bad news in a row.

First of all, Dr Ind called to tell me that I am

41

definitely in stage two cancer and the doctors need to sit down and talk me through it step by step tomorrow. Great!

Then Jack's mum Mary rang me to say that Jack has been sentenced to eighteen months in prison. It felt as though my world fell apart all over again.

He'll only serve half inside and half with an electronic tag, but he is still being taken away from me just when I need him the most. I thought back to when we kissed good-bye that morning and I wished him luck. I didn't believe for a minute I wouldn't be seeing him again a few hours later. Maybe I should have realised it was a serious charge, but I didn't.

Kate had just got back from Afghanistan that morning and I rang her in hysterics.

'What am I going to do without him? How will I do this? I can't cope!'

She tried to calm me down. Usually she can talk me through crap things that happen and make me see it's not so bad. Not this time. I was just screaming and screaming.

In my hour of real need Jack had been snatched away and it hurt so badly.

I drove round to Mary's house and fell into her arms, sobbing. She is completely gutted that her son has ended up in prison. They are a nice family who live in a lovely house and they have no experience of prison at all. It's another world to Mary. She just can't believe it.

'I need his arms around me so much right now,' I sobbed. 'Why did they have to take him away? I love him and so do my boys. I won't cope without him.'

She tried to comfort me but there wasn't

anything she could say or do to make it better. No one could help me that day. I just had to pick myself up and carry on because there is no other option. That's all I can do. Just carry on.

2nd September 2008

I had a meeting with Dr Ind. Jack would usually have been at my side, but instead Mary offered to come in his place.

'Don't worry,' I said—I hate putting people to any trouble—but she insisted.

So we drove off to Harley Street together. It took ages to get there and I was late—as usual.

While I was driving, Jack rang me from prison on my mobile.

'Where are you?' he said.

'I'm still driving,' I replied.

'But you're late!' he cried. 'Come on, Jade, this is important.'

I couldn't believe he'd remembered the exact time of my visit and called up to check I got there. He worries about me so much.

We finally arrived and the doctor got out my records and scans and looked at them seriously, then he leant forward in his big chair to explain to me about the operation and the chemo and the radio I would have to have afterwards.

He said softly, 'At this stage, Jade, I would advise my young patients to make a will.'

A will? Excuse me? When a doctor tells you to make a will it's different from your financial advisor telling you.

My lip started to tremble and I could sense

43

Mary was welling up.

'May I have one of your tissues, please?' I said, reaching for the box.

Then tears started streaming down my face. God, this cancer business was really serious. *Who makes a will at twenty-seven, for god's sake? I shouldn't have to think of such things.*

*   *   *

After the meeting, standing outside in the corridor I started to sob again. 'I might die,' I cried, feeling really low all of a sudden.

Mary put her arm around me. 'No, you won't,' she said. 'You are so strong. You'll get yourself through this.'

I knew she meant well, and I was glad she was there, but sometimes I get sick of being called 'strong'. It's like anything that's chucked at me, I just have to get on with and I'm sick of it. What else could I do but be strong? There were no choices. We walked back to the car park together. 'Can you drive?' I asked, handing her the keys. 'I don't feel able to.'

I could see she was nervous. It was a new £135,000 Bentley, so I understood why.

'You'll be fine,' I said. 'I trust you.'

She got in the car while I went to the ticket machine to pay. It didn't work. So I went to another machine. It didn't work.

I pressed a buzzer to speak to a man. The conversation went something like this:

'Excuse me, could you lift the barrier please?' I asked.

'Sorry?' he said.

'Excuse me, the ticket machine doesn't work, could you lift the barrier?'

'I don't understand you,' he replied. 'Can't help.'

'Please. Can. You. Lift. The. Barrier,' I asked, again.

'No, I don't think I can,' he replied rudely.

This went on for about five minutes. Not only did I have cancer and had been told to make a will, but I was now stuck in an underground car park. At some moment very soon I was going to lose it.

'Excuse me, sir, I am trying to explain, we are stuck in this fucking car park,' I yelled, my voice echoing round the concrete walls.

I could see Mary almost laughing.

Another man came on the line and immediately the gate went up.

Why is nothing ever simple?

We drove home, and I just sat in silence. Thinking, always thinking of my boys and how this cannot, will not beat me.

*   *   *

Back home, I told the boys Jack has gone away to Africa to save the lions. I can't tell them he's gone to prison. That would break their hearts.

He rang later on and we agreed we are going to talk on the phone every day that he is inside. He seems to be dealing with things really well and is just worried about me.

He says he has settled into prison life pretty easily and every day is merging into one.

Hearing his voice gives me strength. Somehow thinking and worrying about him stops me thinking

45

and worrying about myself and all the drugs and treatments I've got coming up.

I'm going to have to take lots of different medicines with horrible side effects to stand a chance.

I tried to think of ways to explain it to the boys that they will understand and decided that I will explain my hair loss, when it happens, by saying I used the wrong shampoo. I could pretend I used that hair-removing stuff by accident.

And I will tell them that I have tadpoles in my belly. A couple of years ago Jack decided to dig a pond in my garden (without asking my permission, I should add!). I was annoyed but he said it would only be a small one and would look nice. Then he some put carp and terrapins in it. I insisted on putting up a gate too because Freddy was only a toddler and could have fallen in.

Anyway, two of the carp died and then one of the terrapins exploded! I don't know what was wrong with it. It just split into white goo and nearly made me and Bobby sick looking at it. Mum reckons it had salmonella, but I'm not sure if terrapins get food poisoning. Anyway, I tried to fish all the yuck out of the pond and then, of course, I fell in! It was horrible. I emerged covered in slime and pondweed. Of course, everyone thought it was hilarious.

So I told the boys that night: 'Remember when Mummy fell in the pond? Well, I swallowed a frog and they made some tadpoles and now they are upsetting Mum's tummy.'

They seemed to understand that. It made perfect sense to them. I hope they don't get frightened of tadpoles, though.

It does make me feel sick to think about my op getting closer.

People have always said to me, 'You're so lucky, Jade!'—and of course I am in some ways. But I always think that just when things are going right for me there has to be some big drama. A lot have been of my own making, of course, but this time is different.

I don't smoke, I eat healthily (lots of fruit and veg), I don't drink every day, I exercise (on and off), I look after myself, I don't do anything wrong and yet I have cancer.

I must be the unluckiest lucky person out there!

3rd September 2008

Mum is back at last and I was really pleased to see her. We sat down and had a cuddle and I told her all the details about my cancer treatments.

'Jade, I know you'll be alright,' she said.

I felt like losing it. '*How* do you know, Mum? Do you understand just how serious this could be?'

Trouble is, I don't think she does. She thinks I am so strong I can get over whatever is thrown at me.

'You'll just have the cells zapped again like you did before,' she said.

'Mum, it's a bit more than that. I might need a hysterectomy,' I said.

'A hyster what?' she replied.

'My womb taken out!' I yelled.

Mum looked into my eyes and could see I wasn't messing.

'Whatever happens I am here for you, Jade,' she

said.

However much we bicker sometimes, it's really good she's around. It's times like this when a girl needs her mum.

Later I spoke to Jack again. He can only ring at 4.30pm so I try to make sure I am in. He's in Chelmsford Prison and says he doesn't want me to visit because it's so grim.

'Prison doesn't bother me,' I said. I knew all about prisons, having grown up visiting my dad in them.

'I just don't want you in this horrible place,' he said.

I am gutted as I'm desperate to see him. Instead we can only talk on the phone. I suppose it's better than nothing and we are getting on better than ever, but it's not the same as being able to kiss and touch him and feel his special hugs.

Having cancer has made us both realise how much we love each other. It would be great if we could get together properly now and stop all the messing about.

4th September 2008

Went shopping with Danielle in Harlow. Just went to the bank and got a few bits.

Suddenly, as I was walking down the street, my left leg went underneath me. It felt all weird, like banging the funny bone in my elbow. Danielle helped me up again.

'What's that about?' I asked, half laughing. She looked really worried.

I've collapsed a few times over the years and the

doctors always said it was nothing. Surely I can't have had this cancer all that time?

*　　　*　　　*

Later on I heard that Katie Price stuck the knife in. We go back a long way and have had our ups and downs but I was shocked about what she said in a magazine interview. 'I feel sorry for anyone who's going through what Jade's going through, but I can't believe she is paid for interviews on subjects that people are really traumatised by . . .' I suppose she is entitled to her opinion but I was upset by it. Surely if I want to talk about my own cancer then it's my decision?

It felt like a right slap in the face. I would never make such comments about someone who has cancer. It's cruel. Anyway, didn't she talk about it when she had a little cancer growth on her finger that her manicurist spotted? I am sure she did.

7th September 2008

Went to Danielle's little girl Rosie's second birthday party with the boys. It was at Dani's mum's house. Little Rosie is such a cutie! Bobby and Freddy love playing with her.

I went there early and helped to fill the party bags and do the sandwiches. Danielle kept saying I didn't have to but I wanted to. I love kids' parties.

When everyone arrived, though, it was full of babies and little girls, which I found hard.

I started feeling all choked up about not having my own little girl. I've always wanted one so I could give her the childhood that I never had, with loads of lovely dresses, and pink stuff . . . she'd be a proper princess. Spoilt rotten. I could relive my childhood again through her.

I was doing okay until a couple turned up with their newborn baby.

I had a peek and said 'Isn't he lovely?' and joined in the oohing and aaahing but inside my heart was cracking into pieces.

Then the dad started saying how great it is to be a dad and all the nice things that come with it— like seeing them when they first wake up in the morning—and that being a father is the best thing that can happen to a man.

It killed me inside to think of Jack never being able to feel that with me.

I couldn't stop myself from welling up again. Danielle spotted this and took me upstairs to calm down.

'Don't hug me,' I said to her. 'Otherwise I will start crying. Stay away.'

'You need to let it out sometimes, Jade,' she said. 'You need to let yourself be sad.'

'I can't do this,' I cried. 'All the kids and babies is too much for me.'

She tried to make me feel better, but it's hard.

'You've got two beautiful sons,' she said. 'Everyone thinks they are gorgeous and they are. I tell you what—you can swap them for Rosie if you like and I am sure you'd want to give her back after a night.'

I managed to laugh.

I sorted myself out a few minutes later and went back to join everyone. I am not ungrateful for my boys. I love them to bits. But I won't be able to build a family with Jack.

I have to let go of my idea of a little girl. She will never exist now.

*　　　*　　　*

When I got home I wanted to take my mind off things, so I decided to focus on DIY. I ripped up the carpet off my floors and painted the oak floorboards white. God, it looked awful.

I rang Kate because she sometimes works on TV home makeover shows. 'Kate, I've just ruined my floors!' I said. 'I need your TV show to come and sort my house out. You can do that while I'm in hospital next week.'

Kate laughed. 'Don't know that we can organise that, Jade, but my mum could help.'

Kate's mum, Lynne, does interior design and she came over to have a look. I flicked through the paint colours she brought and kept changing my mind about what I wanted! It was good to think of something other than operations for once.

I love my house. It's the most expensive thing I've bought but it's the best home I've ever had. It's at the bottom of a narrow tree-lined country lane. At the back are some beautiful rolling fields and it's really quiet. The garden is nice and big for the boys.

It's a whole world away from Bermondsey. My mum still has a flat there and takes the boys to stay sometimes, so they get the best of both worlds. They love London but I think they prefer the peace of our countrysidey [sic] house.

51

Chapter Five

The Operation

9th September 2008

All the preparations for my op start today. I am getting well nervous. Have to have lots of blood test and scans and stuff so they know what's what.

It's a pretty big deal this. I try not to think about it too much. Just concentrating on my DIY! (When I say DIY, obviously I am not doing it myself, but you know what I mean.)

Kate's mum Lynne came over with her friend Claudia to start the work. I've told them I want it to be looking like a palace when I come home from hospital.

I think I've got a good eye for colours— although maybe not when I look at old photos of some of the outfits I've worn over the years . . .

10th September 2008

The boys go to their dad's today. I explained to them first that I need to go into hospital so that the tadpoles in my tummy can be put to sleep. In my book they are far too young to know what the word 'cancer' means and there is no need to tell them.

I am planning to go and see Jack in prison later because I need a cuddle with him before the

52

operation. I can't wait to touch him and see him again. I know he's very worried about me and looking forward to seeing me too.

Then just after lunch I got the worst news: Jack is being moved to a different prison so I can't go today. I had no idea this was going to happen. My whole world just seemed to stop when I found out. I so badly needed to see him. *Why isn't he here?*

I sat and watched TV all evening, depressed and upset but trying not to think about it. I keep smiling and putting on a brave face.

I said on camera, for my Living TV show, that people must think I am not taking this seriously as I laugh and joke about it all the time. But no one is taking it more seriously than me. I'm the mum of two small boys, for god's sake.

This operation is one of the biggest you can have—they say as big as a heart transplant. That is proper scary. If it all goes well, they will only do a radical hysterectomy to cut all the cancer out. We're praying that it hasn't spread beyond the womb.

I've had surgery before (on my boobs) but nothing like this. I wonder what the scar will be like? Don't reckon I'll be buying a new bikini for a while.

11th September 2008

The day of the pre-op. Got up at 6am to clean the house from top to toe. I've never minded cleaning. I am not being tight but why pay someone else to do it when you can do it yourself? I am a house-proud person.

Danielle, Jeff and my mum are going to share the school runs. They've sorted out a rota and they've all got their jobs to do to take care of the boys.

Danielle turned up to help load the car then we picked up Mum at her place. They both kept looking at me, asking me if I was okay. I kept smiling and saying yes.

But I admit that as we got nearer the hospital, my tummy started churning like a washing machine.

When the nurses got the drip set up and took blood from me, I started to panic inside.

'This is a really big thing and it's tomorrow,' I thought.

Dr Coxon came up to see me and somehow managed to make me laugh. She's a nice woman.

I've got lots of fruit in my fridge. Then Charlene popped in to visit and it was so good to see her. She's always around when I need her.

I had a sleeping tablet as I feel very anxious and know I won't sleep, then I sent everyone home.

'We'll stay,' said Mum.

'No,' I said. 'I just need to sleep.'

I needed to be on my own.

12th September 2008

The day of my operation, I woke up so nervous I felt sick. I sent my friends a text:

'Hello everyone, your friend or family member Jade Goody is a little scared as I am about to go down for my op but is a strong girl so please don't worry, love to you all.'

I do want this cancer crap out of my body though. All of it, as soon as possible. Please let it work! Please let that be the case!

Danielle and Mum turned up in time to help me put my operation gown on. They are such embarrassing flapping things, wide open at the back. I'm getting used to doctors seeing my bits now. I can't count how many have examined me down there over the years. Dozens of them!

I'm just trying to be grateful that my womb has already made my lovely boys. Thank God I had them already. It doesn't bear thinking about if I hadn't.

I was scared but insisted on walking myself to the theatre. I refused to have any pre-op medicine because I feel better, as though I am fighting it, when I'm in control. I started crying when I saw those theatre doors and had to say goodbye to my mum and Dani.

As they were getting ready to go, I said to Mum in a deep voice: 'What if they turn me into a man? What if they take off my boobs and put them down below so I end up with massive balls? I could end up being called Jason.'

'Jade, stop messing about,' she laughed.

Danielle smiled. 'Can't believe you, Jade,' she said.

I was asked to count back from ten as they stuck the needle in.

*   *   *

Eight hours later I woke up in intensive care, feeling pretty woozy.

'Am I Jason?' I asked my mum.

55

'No, Jade, your bits are in the same place,' she said.

Danielle gave a little laugh. 'I can't believe you remembered that,' she said.

I slept some more and when I woke up again a niggling pain was hurting my tummy.

Mum told me that she and Danielle had been praying in the hospital chapel. Apparently doctors had said at one point I might need my left leg off if the cancer had spread.

I'm not sure if Mum got that right, but they went to pray it wouldn't happen.

I don't want to look at the scar. They say I'll need to be here for about ten days and no driving for a few weeks afterwards. What am I gonna do without my car? I'm totally dependent on it.

The womb is being tested in the lab at the moment. They think it's good news because they've taken it all out.

All I can do now is rest and get better.

13th September 2008

The staff in this hospital are lovely. I am staying in intensive care for a few days while I wait for the operation results.

I'm missing my boys, though. Mum and Jeff are sharing looking after them. They have a fixed routine with me and I like them to stick to it. It always goes: up for breakfast, lunch around 1 to 2pm, dinner 4.30 to 5.30pm, then bath and bed around 7.30 to 8.30. I am such a routine-loving mum! I stick to it like an army soldier or something. Danielle is the same with Rosie.

When it's bedtime I ignore my phone or whatever else is going on. It's my special time with the boys. They have stacks of books and I read with them every night.

My mum used to get words wrong when she read to me. I remember she kept talking about a 'vinegar car' in one story. I couldn't read well enough myself to know what it was but 'vinegar car' didn't make much sense to me and we had a row about it. In the end I asked my teacher and he said it was a vintage car. Well done, Mum!

When she went on the show *Extreme Makeover* Mum found out she needed her eyes lasered and she could read much better afterwards. Her reading problems before were because she couldn't see!

Dr Ind popped in to say the results are back and I'm definitely gonna need chemo and radiotherapy. That's what we expected. I just have to brace myself for it.

14th September 2008

I asked Danielle to use her camera to take some pictures of me in intensive care.

At first she said no. 'Jade, your mum would go mental if I took pictures of you all wired up like this,' she said. But I talked her into it.

My arms are covered with bruises as they can never find the right veins. It takes them loads of goes with the needle. Ouch!

I want her to record everything for my diary to prove how far I've come afterwards when I am better. I will forget all of this and I want to remember.

I even got Danielle to take a picture of my catheter. She asked if I thought it was a bit much, but I've got no reason to be embarrassed.

People need to know about these things.

17th September 2008

My friend Caroline came to see me. I feel better and am in a good mood. Jack's been transferred to a new prison now, Waylands in Norfolk. Hopefully when I get better I can visit him there. I've chatted to him and he says it's not as bad as Chelmsford.

Mum is taking the boys to her flat soon. She's such a good Nanna. Every time they come over to hers, Bobby always wants to watch *Extreme Makeover* (even though it's a bit gory) and Freddy likes jumping around to the music of my fitness videos (I won't be doing one of them for a while!).

For them it's so normal we are on TV. They probably assume all kids are. It doesn't affect them at all.

18th September 2008

Kate came to visit today with her mum. I quizzed her about the DIY they're doing for me.

'I want it all done for £10K—the windows, the walls, the floors, the lot,' I said.

Kate laughed and said I might need to spend a bit more. She reckons it would cost a bomb to do all that.

It's Freddy's birthday today. He's four years old.

I can't believe it—he's grown up so fast. I hate to miss it. Jeff is taking him to a play area in Epping and then on to a restaurant for a big dinner with his little friends.

It's the first and hopefully the last birthday of theirs I will ever miss.

Mark, my lovely agent, came in for a visit too. I'm booked to appear in a pantomime in Lincoln in December and he's worried I won't be up to it.

'It's so much work and you'll be having chemo at the time,' he said.

I just laughed. 'Honestly, Mark, I'll be fine.'

He knew better than to argue when my mind was made up.

'Okay, let's play it by ear then,' he said.

I told him about my other plans. 'I want my own chat show like Piers Morgan and I want to go to Hollywood next year.'

That would be my dream. It sounds nutty but I know I could do it and the boys would love America.

Mark just told me to focus on getting better first and he'd see what he could do.

20th September 2008

At last the boys came for a visit. I told them that hopefully the tadpoles are not in my tummy any more.

It felt so good to see them and hold their little hands again. They were full of news about everything that was happening at school and all the friends they'd been playing with and I loved listening to them chatting.

59

Kids don't seem to mind hospitals and they were interested in all the machines and what they did.

I was just so happy to be with them again. They made me feel as though this will all be alright. It's got to be, for their sakes.

Chapter Six

Radio and Chemo

24th September 2008

A team of doctors are looking at all my results and scans. The bad news is that, as they feared, they've found a bit of cancer outside the womb and they think I need a whole year of chemo now, after five weeks of radiotherapy.

What a nightmare! I'd hoped this would be done and dusted within a few months. It means it's more serious than they thought.

I had my first dose of radiotherapy today. I had to lie down flat with a paper towel on my bits. It made my skin smell of burning—how horrible is that? A sweet, smoky smell. It doesn't hurt but it feels strange, as if I am in a sci-fi movie.

It only lasted for three minutes. I don't understand how it works. All I know is I have to trust the doctors now. And I do trust these ones here at the Marsden. They seem to know what they're talking about and they tell it to me straight.

26th September 2008

Home at last. Danielle came and picked me up from hospital. She had Rosie in the car with her.

'Sorry, Jade,' she said. 'I couldn't find anyone to look after her.'

I didn't mind at all as I love Rosie. She is such a cutie and cheers me right up.

Bobby and Freddy couldn't stop jumping up and down when I got back. Mum was looking after them.

When I see her with them I do feel proud of her. She's come such a long way from the druggie she was ten years ago. She never did all the things with me that she does with my boys—like giving them individual days. Bobby's day is Saturday, when they go ice-skating or ten-pin bowling, and Freddy's day is Sunday, when he always wants to go and feed the ducks. She is always treating them to the cinema as well.

In fact, my mum is like one big kid herself with her grandchildren. She'll throw eggs at them or go outside and play 'dead' and take ages to wake up. 'Nanna, wake up!' they shout. They love it. She dresses up with them in their fancy-dress costumes. I've walked in on her playing Wonderwoman or Catwoman while Bobby and Freddy are Batman and Robin. She makes me giggle.

She's so close to them both.

I think they bring out the best in her.

I can trust her to make them proper dinners too. Her favourite is chicken and peas with rice. My mum was always into proper home-cooked meals, just as I am.

I spent most of my childhood looking after her or protecting her. We lived in rough areas of Bermondsey and Peckham, and Mum used to use stolen credit cards and chequebooks. She was always drunk or stoned.

I rolled my first joint when I was Freddy's age! Imagine that! Aged four, I also hid her stolen chequebook and credit card stuff in the house during a raid by police.

That was before she got into the harder drugs like crack when I was eighteen.

I'm so glad my boys won't be going through any of that. It's something to tell them when they're older, I suppose. Much older.

Mum is like a different person now. She's always been my mum and I've always loved her, but she is a brilliant granny compared to a mother.

Getting in *BB3* brought me the money that meant my kids want for nothing. They can have a mum who loves them without any of the bad stuff. We can focus on the good things and having fun!

Right now being a good mum isn't easy, though.

I am in my late twenties yet feeling like an old woman, with loads of niggling aches and pains. I do my best to keep up with my boys and put on a brave face, but it's not always easy.

*   *   *

Jack called and I put the boys on to talk to him.

Freddy asked: 'Where are the giraffes? Where are the lions? Where are the snakes? Where are the elephants?' He went through every single animal and talked for ages.

Jack didn't mind, even though it was using up

62

his phone credit. He's so patient with them and loves talking to them. He writes to me and the boys almost every day.

I miss him so much. He is all I could ever want.

30th September 2008

I managed to do the school run today. So pleased for it to be all normal again.

I got the boys up and gave them breakfast (I like them to start with a proper meal like scrambled eggs on toast), then cleaned their teeth with their electric brushes.

It makes me feel good to send them off all smart and clean. They are a couple of beautiful children. My boys are gorgeous!

Simon came and took some snaps of me dropping them off. I've been working with him and Danny since I left the *BB* house in 2002 and I trust them not to take pictures I don't want them to.

I had to go for my usual morning radiotherapy then Danielle persuaded me to go out to lunch. I really didn't want to. I just want to hide at home.

'Not that I want their sympathy but people will think this is not serious if I just go out and have fun.'

'You'll feel so much better for it,' she said. 'Just come.'

So we went to Piano Lounge in Epping and I'm glad I did because it was a giggle. I wore a little dress and dolly shoes. (That's what I call them. I think the real name is Mary Janes.)

'You look amazing,' she said.

It did feel good to dress up a bit and make an

63

effort.

On the way back we bopped around in the car to some house music that we used to go clubbing to.

Afterwards I was so sore. 'I feel like I've been hit with a baseball bat,' I said. My tummy is very tender. I guess you're not supposed to do too much dancing straight after surgery.

I can't believe we used to go out and do that till 6am every weekend years ago. I feel like I'm getting old!

1st October 2008

Mary came with me to hospital to have a port fitted in my chest. This is a small plastic tube that's put under my skin and that is where the chemo drugs will go. It makes my skin crawl just thinking about it. I hate this.

I had to have an anaesthetic as they did it and when I woke up I wanted Jack.

'Where is he?' I asked, a bit wandered.

'I'm here instead,' said Mary. 'Don't worry, we're going to see him at the weekend.'

I started crying as I touched the port in my chest. It feels so horrible and weird.

'They've taken my arm off,' I cried.

'No,' said Mary, gently. 'You're confused. It's just in your chest.'

It has to stay with me until the first lot of chemo is finished in four weeks' time. It feels like it is taking over my body. I don't want a piece of tube stuck inside me near my heart. It's going to be a constant reminder than I am ill.

2nd October 2008

Have a shoot for *OK!* today but first I'm getting my hair cut. I've always liked messing with my hair and have had it chopped off before. This time feels different, though, because it's for a terrible reason. My chemotherapy is going to make it fall out so the nurses advised me to cut it first because it might mean I can keep it for longer.

I reckon I'll get used to it. I just feel upset to be forced into it.

I rang Danielle to tell her. She once said she didn't like my hair short.

'I'll cut mine off too then,' she said straight away.

'Don't be stupid,' I said, then I started crying. *No womb and now short boys' hair.* 'I don't feel I've got my femininity any more,' I sobbed.

Danielle tried to cheer me up. 'If you have to have it shaved then so will I,' she said. 'And chances are yours will grow back and mine won't!'

That's the next thing to think about—no hair at all! I would look like a rugby player. Or an egg with massive lips.

I'll try not to let it get me down.

I met Mark outside the flat in West London where we were to meet the hairdresser but when I saw the guy I nearly had a heart attack! His hair looked like he'd stuck a finger in a light socket. I'm sure it's the new style—but blimey! Did I really want him anywhere near mine?

I didn't want to offend him though so I let him get on with the cut. I couldn't look at Mark, who kept making me laugh as if he knew what I was thinking.

Afterwards I went into the bathroom with Mark, looked at myself in the mirror and burst into tears.

'This is it,' I said. 'It's starting . . .'

'Well, at least it looks better than the hairdresser's,' he said.

'Thanks,' I smiled. That's why I like Mark—he's not full of bullshit.

I went to Danielle's mum's house afterwards with the boys. She does brilliant dinners. I love her food.

'Your hair looks nice,' Danielle's brother Luke said straight away.

'Don't take the piss, you,' I said.

'I mean it,' he replied.

'Did you hear me? I said: "Don't take the flipping piss!"'

Everyone laughed. He'd better mean it!

Every time I pass a mirror, I keep looking at myself trying to get used to it. *What will Jack think? I hope he doesn't hate it.*

5th October 2008

I visited Jack for the first time at Wayland Prison in Norfolk. He didn't want any visitors up until now because he was too upset. He is quite a proud person in some ways and doesn't want me to see him locked up.

I went with his mum and dad, Mary and Andy.

I've been to prisons before when I was visiting my dad. He was convicted for drugs and thieving and stuff so many times and spent most of his life in prison. I remember visiting him after I got

66

famous in *BB* and I was so chuffed we took a picture together. Of course, our new-found relationship didn't last long as he sold the snap for loads of money to the tabloids. He never changed! Later on he asked for a picture of Bobby. I bet he sold it and used the money to buy drugs. That was the last straw for me.

Then he died of a heroin overdose in 2005. He was found slumped in a Kentucky Fried Chicken toilet in Bournemouth next to a needle. What a way to go! He was only forty-two, for god's sake. I didn't go to his funeral because he chose drugs over me and I could never forgive him for that.

As I said, I do feel a bit different now. I will probably go to his grave and lay some flowers to make peace. He probably did the best he could.

At the prison, Mary was a bit nervous and kept pinching herself so as not to cry.

'You'll be okay,' I said. 'It's not that bad. Come on.'

We walked through security and had dogs sniffing round us. That brought back memories. Because my dad went inside for drugs we were always thoroughly searched. I remember as a kid being searched as I visited my dad in prison. It was horrible. I was scared I was going to be thrown in the cells.

All this was routine stuff, but I felt for Mary. She was so upset her son was in here.

I just couldn't wait to see Jack. We all sat round a table and Andy cried, the tears dripping down his face. Of course it's not nice to see your son in the nick. I'd be devastated if it was Bobby or Freddy (not that it ever will be—they are good boys!).

After a bit of chitchat they left Jack and me

alone. He looked all pale because he'd not been on a sunbed for six weeks.

Holding his hand was brilliant. I miss him so much and so do my boys.

They keep talking about Jack's visit to the jungle. Bobby wants to go and visit him there. Jack's even written them some really sweet letters talking about his jungle life.

'How are you, babe?' he asked.

I tried not to talk about the cancer because people were all around us and there was no privacy, but it was hard.

'You'll be okay,' he said, trying to be positive.

I know Jack hasn't been inside before but I'm sure he'll be fine. A few of my old school friends from Bermondsey are in there with him (for robbery, possession of firearms and so on) and are looking out for him. Some people my mum knows are also in there. That's coming from a Bermondsey estate for you!

Sitting at that table made me want a hug from him so badly but we were only allowed to hold hands. At least it's not as bad as the time I visited my dad in prison and there was a glass wall between us.

Before we left, I promised to write as much as possible. We are going to speak on the phone every day around 4pm. Jack will try and ring my home phone as he doesn't have much credit for mobiles.

It was hard to go and I shed a few tears on the way back, but at least I could see for myself that he was okay. If he behaves himself he'll be out in January some time and that's not too far away, I suppose.

6th October 2008

It's a two-hour drive every morning to my radiotherapy for a session that only lasts three minutes, and sometimes it seems like a waste of time—but those three minutes could save my life.

When I arrive, the nurses have to make sure it's in exactly the same spot each time. I am glad I don't have to work it out myself! It is clever what they do and I am learning a lot. I just lie on a couch with a paper towel over my bits while the machine whirls round me.

It feels a bit tingling at first. Afterwards it makes my tummy gurgle like a drain.

One of the real downers is that I'm not allowed hot baths any more because radiotherapy makes your skin sensitive. You try relaxing in a cold bath! It's such a shame as I love my baths with tons of smelly oils.

The press have been saying I've contacted all these famous people who've had cancer, like Kylie or Trisha, but in all honesty I haven't. I'm in the public eye but I have almost no celebrity friends. All my friends are just normal people who go to work. I ring them up when I'm crying. I ring them up when I'm happy. I know there are some people who only want to hang out with celebrities but I'm not like that at all. And why would I call complete strangers to talk about my cancer? Pul-lease!

9th October 2008

Radiotherapy and then my first chemo session today. Kevin Adams came with me. He was my personal trainer when I left the *BB* house. He knew my agent at the time and was given the (difficult) job of getting me in shape.

I was terrified of Kevin at first because he is a really huge guy, but I needed someone tough like him to push me on at our training sessions.

Anyway, we stayed in touch and because my other friends have normal nine-to-five jobs they can't help do hospital runs. Kev works freelance so he insists on helping when I can't manage. I don't usually like people coming in case I just want to sleep, but Kev doesn't seem to mind.

An interview has just come out that I did with *OK!* magazine in which I talked about my funeral plans, so we were chatting about that cheery subject! I said I wanted to have an open funeral and let everyone who wanted to come along. I want people to cry over me!

And I don't want people to have a booze-up because I think getting drunk at funerals is a bit disrespectful. They can have a cup of tea instead. Not that I think it's going to come to that. I'm still planning to beat this thing.

When the nurses started hooking up the chemo bag to a drip into my arm and putting the blue bag over the top so the light won't get to it, I thought: *'Oh my god, this is real. These drugs are strong.'*

I started crying and Kev got a bit upset then, too, but it wasn't so bad. At least it didn't hurt.

First I had to have bags and bags of saline fluid and drugs put through me to 'flush' me out. It's horrible because even though it's supposed to make my body better I know it's going to make me feel ill. It will take six hours to pass into my body. That's a long time to sit about.

Once a month for the next twelve months I have to have two types of chemo drugs pumped into me through a tube.

I got my phone and took a photo of myself with all the tubes and bags and sent it to Mark, suggesting he could put it out there to show the world this cancer is the real thing.

He called back and said, 'No way, Jade!'

Kevin decided to head off for a bit while I had the treatment but he couldn't find our car! He came back up to say there was glass on the floor and he thought it had been stolen. I was worried about him so I walked all the way downstairs, carrying my chemo drip. I shouldn't have left the room but I wanted to find out what had happened and no nurses were watching. The squeaky wheels on the drip sounded like a horror film noise echoing down the corridor.

I found Kev downstairs looked mugged off. He was a bit surprised to see me.

'What you doing here?' he asked.

'I was worried,' I said.

'Don't worry about this!' he said. 'Just worry about yourself!'

Turns out we'd got a ticket and a car clamp too. How much bad luck is that?

I started laughing at the look on Kev's face and it cheered me up a bit.

I was sick soon after that, but thought: 'Oh well, it's not that bad.'

Afterwards I let the photographers waiting

outside get a shot of me holding the parking ticket. What do you think the chances are that they'll let us off the fine?

10th October 2008

I had a long chat with Jack.

He said he always asks people what they are in for (which you're not supposed to do) and he gets upset sometimes, as some of them have done awful things, like murders.

Poor Jack. He tells me he can handle himself, but I worry a bit.

'Just keep yourself to yourself,' I tell him.

I keep writing him letters and sending in photographs of us and the boys. It must be so boring sitting in that cell all day. I would go completely mental if it was me.

11th October 2008

The boys are away with Jeff this weekend. I suddenly felt full of energy and rang Mary to see what she was doing.

'We're off to a wedding show in Battersea Park,' she said.

Jack's sister Laura is getting married in September next year so I thought I'd go along and soak up the ideas!

When we arrived I didn't have a ticket, but I told them my agent had put me on the guest list and they let me in.

People there were so nice. I had loads coming

up to me, saying, 'Good luck, Jade!' One lady came and gave me a hug, asking 'How are you feeling?'

Truth is, I do feel good today.

The fashion show was amazing and I especially loved the Pronovias dresses.

'You wait till I tell Jack about this!' I laughed to Mary.

I've told her in confidence that having cancer has made me realise I want to marry Jack but that it is up to him to ask me. I know she is all for it.

We got loads of free samples. Laura was taking notes for her big day. She spotted some beautiful napkins all folded nicely.

'Do you like those?' I asked.

'Yes,' she said, so I picked one up and popped it into my bag.

'You can't do that,' said the lady.

I hadn't realised it was part of the display!

We had champagne and sushi for lunch and it was a lovely day out, thinking about positive, happy things. I think it did me a lot of good.

12th October 2008

I feel more determined than ever today.

I will not be a cancer victim.

I will not let cancer get the better of me.

I will always get the better of cancer.

I will always be stronger than it.

There's a cancer cell and there's me and I will always be stronger than the cancer cell because I need to live.

I really do think I am going to get better now.

I've heard that positive thinking helps and no one could be more positive than me.

Chapter Seven

'I'm Working On It'

15th October 2008

Opened Homme Fatal today in partnership with a mate of mine called Julie who's already got a salon in Loughton, Essex, called Femme Fatale.

I know it's hard to believe but people do say I have a good business brain! I'm a silent partner this time. I'd already had a go at running my own salon, Ugly, but it closed as I didn't have enough time to spend on it. I've done a beauty course and learned to do things like waxing la-las and eyebrow plucking—all very useful for my posse of girls (if they ever let me near them).

I'm also planning on opening my own boot camp next year. I teamed up with a beautician and health person called Nilam Patel who is going to run it with me. We've come up with a whole package of training and good food, and girls can go there to trim up and have some fun. I've lost two stone on one before so I know they work! It's well-known that I've been a yo-yo dieter over the years so I can relate to anyone else who struggles with their weight. Hopefully we'll have lots of bookings and I'll pop down to help out when I can.

The opening has been postponed until January, when I'm crossing my fingers that I will be better and able to open it myself. For now, Nilam will keep it all ready and waiting for me.

It's good to have so much in the pipeline. Things are going well on that score. I've done alright so far as Jade, but I want to start my own empire. I think people who inherit money are lucky but it's not the same as building it up yourself. I want to sell it all when it's worth loads of money and then retire at thirty-five and enjoy myself.

I am proud of what I've done but it could be bigger still!

Also, hopefully everything will be alright, but if it's not then at least the boys will benefit from all this. Even when I'm feeling positive and optimistic there's always a bit of a shadow in the background.

16th October 2008

Chemo again. Mum came with me today. She would come more often but she can't drive because of her dead arm. She tucks the hand in her pocket to keep it out the way. It was really bad luck that she lost the use of her left hand when she is left-handed!

Today I walked into the wrong hospital room and saw lots of women breastfeeding. That reminded me that I'll never have another baby or my little girl and I got a bit upset. All of a sudden it just hits you, like a punch in the gut.

Mum gave me a hug. 'You know your boys will make up for it,' she said. 'They might even have girls themselves one day and you'll have grand-daughters.'

I started to feel better.

'But,' she continued, 'That baby you lost when you had the miscarriage was probably a little girl anyway, so you weren't supposed to have her . . .'

'Mum!' I screamed. 'Only you could come up with something like that. You're supposed to be making me feel better not worse!'

She doesn't half put her foot in it sometimes. There are no prizes for guessing where I get it from.

She looked a bit upset. 'Sorry, I didn't mean it.'

I rang Kev straight away to tell him. 'You'll never believe what my mum just said . . .' He was horrified, of course!

I feel rough today. I look like Henry the Hedgehog with this hairdo. I can't do anything with it because it's not long enough for hairclips even.

17th October 2008

I met up with Max, Mark and Living TV to talk about my TV show. Originally I'd wanted to get better before starting filming again but my treatment is going to last for months and I need the money to support my boys. The papers are full of details about my cancer, whether I talk about it or not, so I might as well have the cancer stuff on my show. We agreed that they will follow me around as I have my cancer treatments. I don't mind showing it. I've already done several successful TV shows, including *Jade's PA* and *Jade's Salon* and had already started filming *Live with Jade*.

The last production team had to stop filming when I went to India. It's going to start up again now with a new production team and I think it might help me. I want someone special to film it, though—my good friend Kate.

She had been the producer on *Jade's Salon* in 2005 and I trusted her. I knew that if I pooed myself she would turn the camera off and help me. She would make sure I always looked ladylike. I didn't want to do it with someone new, someone I didn't know. I needed Kate from my Fab Four.

They all agreed she could do it, which was a huge relief.

Mark thinks this is a great opportunity to get back into the swing. TV needs a bit of Jade Goody, he said!

It's funny because I am so aware of how this works. If you are not seen to be working and doing well then no one wants you. It's as simple as that. I've not worked much over the last year after all that Shilpa stuff. People said my career was finished, that *Big Brother* made me and *Celebrity Big Brother* broke me.

This is a chance to work properly again. Things are on the up!

19th October 2008

I got my eyebrows tattooed in Milton Keynes today in preparation for when my hair falls out. Seemingly I'll lose the eyebrows and maybe my eyelashes as well. I'll look weird without them and I don't want the kids to get a fright.

I think the tattoos look great, like they're

painted on or something. I'll have to call them no-brows! Got some shots done with them for the papers.

Apparently Kerry Katona has stuck up for me in the Katie Price row. She told the *Daily Mail* online that Katie is totally wrong on this one. 'Jade has already saved many lives with her tireless charity work and the more she sends that important message of cancer awareness, she deserves nothing but credit.'

Aww, that is so nice of her.

23rd October 2008

Mary came with me for my chemo session but first we had breakfast at Carluccio's in South Kensington, which was lovely. We just looked like two normal people having breakfast, not as if we were about to go for cancer treatment.

I cried when they stuck the needle in the port this time. Can you imagine having a needle anywhere near your heart? Somehow it's not right.

The chemo doesn't hurt but it makes me feel really sick afterwards. I get hungry but everything I eat tastes like metal and I throw it up.

I sting all over as if stinging nettles are on my skin. It's just supposed to make my la-la area itchy but I end up itching everywhere—on my head, ears, all over.

Kate has been told that they're not allowed to film the actual chemo sessions for Living TV. The hospital say it's not safe. I wouldn't have minded actually, but it's up to them.

26th October 2008

I stayed at Mary's house last night. I love being here and having dinners cooked for me by Andy, Jack's dad. He's a great cook. I couldn't believe it tonight when he told me the mushrooms I was eating were wild and that he went out and picked them himself.

I wouldn't trust myself to do it in case I got the poisonous ones. Then I began to wonder if Andy was maybe trying to poison me. You never know!

We're visiting Jack tomorrow and his little brother Louis, who's eighteen, is coming along. He's so sweet, like a younger version of Jack, and we have a right laugh.

I knew it wasn't going to be nice for him to see his older brother in jail, so I tried to be supportive.

We got up early and drove to Norfolk. When we arrived the doors were shut so I said to the guards: 'Excuse me but we have a prison visit.'

They laughed. We thought visiting was 7.30am and it was actually at 8.30am. Plus, one of them pointed out that the clocks had gone back and it was only 6.30am! What a bunch of doughnuts we are! There's not a lot to do in Norfolk at that time of the morning, so we went to see Mary's sister-in-law Jenny, who lives nearby, and had a cup of tea.

My tummy was giving me gip again—real cramping pains.

At last we got to see Jack and he was looking okay. He seems to be handling it well.

'I just want to break out and help you,' he said.

'Bad idea,' I told him. 'They'd find you pretty

79

quickly because they can easily find out where I am with my lifestyle at the moment: radiotherapy every morning and chemo every Thursday. It wouldn't take much detective work.'

I told him I was fine and time would soon pass. And it will.

27th October 2008

Living TV started filming me today. I trust Kate and Jill (who does the camera) so much that I don't hold back! As soon as that camera switches on I like having a laugh.

Kate filmed me getting in the bath today.

She said: 'Why don't you drop your dressing gown like Lara Croft?'

'Lara who?'

'You know, the *Tomb Raider* bird.'

'Okay.' And I did it, trying to be sexy but giggling at the same time!

Kate filmed it three times and I was getting fed up. Angelina Jolie needn't worry about the competition after all.

It helps having a camera on me. It keeps me focused. I'm not embarrassed to talk about anything. In fact, I feel better when I talk about things.

I had a chat with Kate in the bath but she let me look at the edits and we erased the film where you could see my nipples and made sure you can't see any of my bits. I want to keep some dignity!

Being so young and being told that I've got something I have no control over has changed me. I don't care any more what people think about me

80

or how they judge me. If I want to talk in the bath, I will.

The boys flew off to Cyprus today with Jeff and his girlfriend Amy for half-term week. I know they'll have a great time but I'm glad I had the filming to distract me.

I hope they have fun—I'm sure they will. Jeff is a good father to them whatever problems we've had in the past.

We met in 2003 and I was very much in love with him but we always had our ups and downs. He was a reality TV star in the show *Shipwrecked*, and before that he had played football for Leyton Orient but left due to injury.

We split up a few times and got back together again, but we split for good when I was three months pregnant with Freddy. It was really tough at the time but I had no choice—I had to carry on.

But the hardest bit is missing my boys when they go off to spend time with their dad. My house feels so big and empty when they disappear.

I am glad in a way this time because I'm having another chemo treatment this week and I don't have to worry about who's looking after them while I'm stuck in a hospital bed.

28th October 2008

Some of the papers ran pictures yesterday of Mum supporting me as I walked out of the hospital. I can't figure out when they were taken, but when I saw them I felt so sad. I looked like total shite and was crying, my hair all sticking up, hobbling along in a tracksuit top. I don't want my boys to see this shot.

I know the paps hang around outside the hospital taking pictures and usually I don't mind. They just have a job to do like everyone else. I've put myself in the public eye, so why not?

These pictures really brought it home to me just how bad things are, though. My mum looks terrible as well—really worried.

Then it struck me that if anything good is to come of this, it's me getting closer to her. She's been like a rock for the last couple of months. All those times in the past when I've looked after her while she was drunk or taking drugs meant she was more like my kid. Finally we've almost got a proper mother and daughter relationship because she's proving she can be there for me.

Kate drove me to hospital for my radiotherapy today. Afterwards I felt really low and had to lie down on the car seat. My bones were killing me and I couldn't stop the tears.

I just didn't feel good at all. I felt like I'm not a woman any more. I felt so sorry for myself and I hate feeling like that.

Kate said, 'Let's go somewhere nice for a treat.'

My first thought was that I fancied a spa treatment so I rang Champneys in Henlow Grange and said: 'You've got to help me.'

We drove there for the afternoon. I was hoping for a proper massage but they said I couldn't have one in case it made the cancer spread. Instead I had a body butter treatment. I got into a right muddle with the towel as they filmed me on the massage bench. I was half-naked with just a G-string on. Someone could have helped me!

A nurse asked me if I wanted reflexology. 'Is

82

that when someone hits you with a stick?' I asked.

Kate was cracking up and that set me off.

I know I get things wrong quite a lot and make people laugh. I know I am not the brightest spark in the book or the sharpest kinfe in the drawer, or whatever it is, but I guess my sense of humour carries me through.

When it was time to leave, I wanted to keep my white Champney's dressing gown.

'You can't,' said Kate. 'Take it back. It's stealing.'

'No,' I grinned. 'I'm keeping it. Just watch me.'

I didn't bother to put my clothes on but walked to the car in it with Kate huffing and puffing at me.

I just laughed at her.

Then after we set off down the motorway, Kate said: 'Hey, good job you don't have to get out of the car . . .'

The cheeky cow didn't tell me I needed petrol, did she?

We had to pull over in a petrol station and I was so embarrassed.

'I've just had radiotherapy and I've got cancer, you can't make me walk about outside with just a dressing gown on,' I wailed. 'It's not fair! People will look at me like I'm a nutter!'

Kate was pissing herself laughing. I had to get out and fill the car up, standing in my dressing gown, freezing my bits off.

Then she felt guilty so she went and paid in the shop.

A day that started so low finished with us on a high because of our lovely pampering session. You can always find something cheerful if you try.

Chapter Eight

How Low Can You Go?

30th October 2008

I've got another dose of chemo booked in for today. I felt so low when I woke up. It's all starting to catch up on me.

The boys weren't here and I've sent Mum home for a break in her flat in Bermondsey.

I suppose being on my own makes horrible thoughts crowd in.

The cancer seems more real.

I'm going to start having the man's hormone testostrom [testosterone] put into my body to give me more energy soon. It's going to be a patch on my arm. I hope it doesn't turn me into a man! I've already got enough of that in the house anyway with two little men of my own.

I sat up and cried for a while, then the phone rang. It was Kate waiting outside with the camera to start filming. I didn't want to answer the door.

'I don't want to do it today,' I cried. 'I want to be alone.'

I've cut myself off from my friends for a while now. I don't invite people round the way I used to. I don't call them. I know Danielle has found it hard, as we were always together before.

Now I didn't want to let the TV crew in either. I am used to dealing with problems on my own. In a way I feel more vulnerable asking for help than if I just handle things myself.

84

'Open the door, Jade,' she said. 'Let us help you.'

I hesitated. I want everyone to go away but then I need to do this filming, and Kate usually makes me feel better. When I opened the door she held out the microphone wire in her hand.

'Do you want to do this?' she asked, looking worried.

I clipped it on automatically—I've done it so many times before with the number of documentaries I've done—and then burst into tears.

'I can't go through with this. I'm so sore and it's horrible,' I cried. 'I just want it all to be over. I don't want it.'

Kate rubbed my hand.

Danielle rang then and when she heard my voice she said she was coming over.

'No, don't,' I cried. I so badly wanted to be left on my own—but she ignored me. Minutes later she was at the door with little Rosie and just seeing her adorable face cheered me up.

'Are you poorly?' Rosie asked me, frowning.

'Yes,' I replied, trying not to cry. 'I have tadpoles in my tummy and the doctors give me magic medicine to take it away.'

Bless her heart, she soon made me smile again.

Kate was pointing at her watch. 'It's 10am and your appointment is for now. Come on, Jade, you have to fight this.'

I knew I was late. Part of me didn't care. *I don't want any more hospital visits. I want it all to go away.*

Kate said again. 'Jade, we have to go.'

I took a deep breath. 'Come on, let's go then.' I

grabbed my keys.

*   *   *

But at the hospital they did some tests and told me I was too ill to have chemo today. Instead they gave me a painkilling drug, which I had a reaction to. I started chucking up in a cardboard bowl. It was so embarrassing. Kate stood in front of me so the Living TV people couldn't see.

Poor Kate is seeing all of this illness right close up.

I felt so ill I asked the hospital if I could stay in for a few days. They can control the pain and it makes me feel safe here. I want to hide away for a bit and get looked after.

I rang Mum and she says she'll look after the boys when they get back and Kevin says he'll do the school run. I am so grateful for their support.

It won't be for long. I will start back as soon as I can . . .

*   *   *

I have a favourite room in the Marsden where I sometimes sit as the chemo treatment is going in. Outside the window there's a beautiful tree. I often look at it. The leaves are starting to change colour, going all orangey for autumn.

'See that tree?' I told myself. 'I've seen it change colour and by the time all the four seasons have passed I will be better again.'

86

31st October 2008

The boys will be away until the 2nd of November but Mum doesn't want them to miss Halloween so she's planning to do it late. She's gone to town buying loads of stuff for when they get back— spiders, a web, witches' stuff, everything. She showed it to me when she came to visit. My sons don't go without!

2nd November 2008

I'm still in the Marsden but when the boys got back they rang to tell me all about their holiday in Cyprus.

They went to a disco every night, swam in a freezing swimming pool, went on a speedboat and to a circus.

Freddy kept pouring himself too much Coca-Cola but Jeff watered it down otherwise he wouldn't sleep! He made friends with a thirteen-year-old girl too—gosh, I wonder if he's got the charm with the ladies already?

I'm glad they got away from all this and had some fun. In one way they're lucky their parents have split up as they get more holidays.

I'm sad to have missed out. Jeff said they all slept with their beds pushed together. It's lovely for them to be so close to their dad.

Oooh, I can't wait to give them the biggest hug. Soon, I hope.

3rd November 2008

I was talking to Danny and Simon about the idea of us going away with the boys. I want to go somewhere hot and forget about all of this. I love the South of France or Spain and fancy going there maybe.

But looking back, as much as I adore my friends, holidays with them are often disastrous.

I managed to singe my hair in a New York hairdressers' (nothing I couldn't sort out with some nail clippers), twist my knee and have to get airlifted by helicopter off a mountain in Morzine, France, and have a big row with Jack before he bashed in my hotel-room door in Marbella. Not even a holiday can be simple in my life. It's a wonder any of my friends want to go away with me. I suppose holidays with me are never boring!

I'm feeling well looked after. It gives me some security being here in the Marsden.

4th November 2008

I'm twenty-seven years old and I'm having hot flushes like a fifty-year-old.

My periods have stopped and I don't feel like a woman any more. I still have my ovaries, but the treatment is killing everything inside them. Chances are nothing can be used.

I'm crying one minute, then I'm hot. I'm all over the place.

It's really frightening. It hasn't hit me properly yet. Every now and then a little bit does, like when I had the first chemo and burst into tears, or when

I had my hair cut. But the whole death thing just can't happen as I need to be here for my kids.

*   *   *

They've told me I've got a 50 per cent chance of living and a 50 per cent chance of dying. It is literally split down the middle. *That is not good odds when it comes to something that is as serious as life or death.*

I didn't know anything about cancer when this all started. I've learned a lot since.

Maybe other people reading this will think: 'Well, if she's going through it maybe it ain't so bad.'

I keep doing interviews because at the end of the day they pay money and that's the least I can do for my children. Every penny gets banked for them and it makes me feel as though I am achieving something just in case I get the wrong 50 per cent and the worst happens.

5th November 2008

I'm still in hospital. My new sofa was being delivered and I called Mum and Kevin to tell them to be there.

Mum says she will be doing a little fireworks display for the boys. I started crying. I am gutted to miss it. Every year she treats them to fireworks, spending about £200 on massive boxes.

I lay in bed tonight listening to all the pops and bangs outside my hospital window, thinking of Bobby and Freddy and all those other kids out there having fun.

I hate this, it's so unfair. I should be at home with them, not stuck in a hospital bed, missing out. It's one of my favourite times of year.

But then none of this is fair. Who ever said life had to be fair? That's not part of the deal at all.

6th November 2008

I came home from hospital today, feeling a bit better and well rested. The staff there are so good. I've started to chat to people and get to know them a bit—like Roy, a guy I see at my radiotherapy most days. We share the same machine.

So many people are going through this. I left with a huge bag of about ten different kinds of tablets. It's so confusing. The doctor said: 'Only take these two kinds if you are in pain.'

But I'm usually in pain so I looked at him and said: 'Well, does that mean I take them or not?' I just don't get it. I don't want to take the wrong ones or more than I need to.

It was freezing outside when we left. Kate came and picked me up and lent me her Louis Vuitton bag to carry all my stuff.

On the way back I said I wanted some sushi because I was fed up with hospital food.

We stopped at a place near Harvey Nicks where I stuffed myself and then felt sick. It was lovely though.

A cameraman called Richard was telling me about some herbal remedy he'd heard of that apparently cures cancer. It sounded like rubbish to me. I don't think I'll be rushing to try it.

* * *

The boys ran to the door as soon as I got home. 'Mummy, shut your eyes,' they said, grabbing my hand.

'Keep them shut!' shouted Freddy as they led me upstairs to their bedroom.

They had written 'Welcome home Mummy!' in chalk on their blackboard.

Mum had obviously done a great job looking after them for me.

'I'm glad you're back,' she said to me. 'The house comes alive when you walk in the door.'

9th November 2008

I took the boys to a firework display at their school today. It was cold and raining so I took off my Prada coat and laid it on the ground for the boys to sit on, then put up an umbrella.

Mum went mad. 'Jade, you're ill and you're standing there in just a bleeding T-shirt! You must be freezing!'

'As long as the boys are alright, so am I,' I said.

They're the best thing in my life. Where would I be without them?

10th November 2008

Guess what? I have a whole three weeks off my treatment! I feel like having a party to celebrate. No hospitals for me for a while.

Whooooopeeeeee!

After that I will have to start my stronger doses of chemo. They will be less regular but they are ones that will take my hair off. It's all swings and roundabouts with this illness. Up one day and down the next.

12th November 2008

I decided to cut Mum's hair today and the Living crew came to film it. As they arrived I was on the phone to the bank because they had cancelled some of my direct debits while I was in hospital.

God, those bankers on the phone drove me flipping mad!

'This is Miss Jade Goody,' I had to scream. 'You have got my money!'

They spoke me like I was some kind of nutter.

After I got it sorted, I sat Mum down to do her hair but she went mental when she saw what scissors I wanted to use.

'They're for pruning roses!' she screamed.

I call them my vegetable scissors as I use them for chopping veg, but they are the best ones in my house.

I remember when Mum had long hair (she was a Rastafarian for nineteen years) and I used nail scissors on it then. It still came out alright.

This time we had a row as I was cutting. The menopause makes me get moody sometimes.

'Right,' I shouted at her when I'd cut one half of her hair. 'Just forget it then!'

'Jade,' shouted Mum. 'Stop taking fucking liberties. Go and get your tablets and calm yourself down. I am NOT going out with half a haircut.'

I finally calmed down and finished it. And it looked great. I gave her a nice bob and dyed it dark brown. Mum was actually really pleased in the end.

I feel so much closer to her these days. Before I probably would just have stormed off and left her with a funny hairdo!

13th November 2008

Got up early as usual to take the boys to school. It's one of my biggest fears not being able to do the school run any more. I like getting them all ready, making sure they are smart and then getting them in on time.

I had a big pile of ironing to do then I went shopping in Bicester Shopping Village with Mary and a friend of hers called Anne Marie. I feel closer to Jack when I hang out with his family.

It was fun. I nipped into Links when they weren't looking and bought them both some sparkly Christmas decorations. I gave Mary a gold Christmas pudding that will match the colour scheme in her front room and Anne Marie got a little house.

'When you put them on your tree every year, think of me,' I said.

Suddenly they both looked a bit pale. 'No, you're going to be fine . . .' stammered Mary. They knew what I was trying to say.

'Please,' I said, before heading off to another shop. I did most of my Christmas shopping while we were there that day. There were loads of bargains.

Jack's dad Andy made us dinner when we got home, then I chatted to his brother Louis and watched TV. I like being part of this normal family. If Jack would just propose to me I could be a proper part of it one day.

Chapter Nine

Finding the Fun

14th November 2008

Boring day sorting out bank stuff and looking at piles of paperwork. It all had to be done and I need to catch up. I can't keep up with it all.

I have people to help me with the business side of things. You know, I've had a lot of ribbing for being thick but Mark tells me I have a great business brain! It just proves you don't need loads of Maths GCSEs to understand what works. I guess I have lots of ideas, even if some of them don't always turn out the way I want them to.

Spoke to Jack. He rang up and his friends were all singing down the phone, pissed off their heads.

'How come you've been drinking?' I asked.

He laughed. 'Home-made hooch.'

Apparently the boys made a special prison brew. They took some orange juice that had gone off and added loads of sugar and left it on the pipes in the prison to heat up for five days. Jack says it doesn't taste very nice but does the job! Sounds disgusting to me. Definitely not one to try at home.

I hope he doesn't get into trouble.

17th November 2008

Another hospital visit for tests and stuff.

Did a face-to-face interview with the Living team: 'I keep saying this but I am bigger and better than cancer and will stamp on this thing and beat it.' I just came out with it and they thought it sounded good.

I bought the boys some new board games. I love Kerplunk. I remember playing it myself. It makes such a racket when you pull out the wrong stick and all the balls fall down. We had a giggle later playing game after game. I think I've lost my touch though because they were beating me every time!

18th November 2008

Jack's got a job in prison cleaning the hallway and he gets paid £9 a week. He says it's so long it's like looking down the M25.

'Hope you do it properly,' I said.

'I just throw water on it and give it a quick mop,' he told me. I don't think I'll be giving him the job of mopping my floors in that case.

All his days are merging into one and speeding past now. He says he still misses me and the boys loads.

'I just want to be there with you,' he said.

I write to him almost every day and he writes back. *I need him so much.*

I got such a big lump in my throat I could hardly

speak. Although maybe I shouldn't talk about having more lumps when I have cancer—don't want to tempt fate.

20th November 2008

Doing a *Love It* magazine photoshoot today for their Christmas issue but Mark has told me not to talk about Christmas because he's already done a deal for an *OK!* Christmas special. Then they turned up with loads of Christmas presents for the shoot. I didn't want to offend anyone, but I tried my best to avoid talking about Christmas while looking at all these gift-wrapped parcels.

Bobby and Freddy were with me, but Bobby was in a mood all day. He's a sensitive soul and he knows I'm fighting this horrible illness. Freddy's too young to take it on board properly but Bobby gets a bit down sometimes and then at other times he gets stroppy. Which is fair enough, actually. I'm doing the same myself.

Then the seamstress from the Lincoln panto showed up with my costume for me to try on for some publicity pictures. I'm playing the part of the wicked 'Queen Tabloid' in their version of *Snow White*. Why do I always get wicked roles? Is someone trying to tell me something?

Bobby was bored while all this was going on and started acting up even more so I asked for the Living TV cameras to be turned off. I got confused and thought they were still filming when they weren't, so I got the hump with them.

I ended up having a row with Kate. 'I thought you were supposed to be straight with me,' I yelled. 'I thought I could trust you. Do you know what? Just forget it!'

I grabbed the boys and we stormed out and jumped in my car to go home.

About half an hour later I got to the end of my road and ran out of petrol. There was only one person to ring.

'Kate?' I said, embarrassed. 'You know, I might need your help . . . I'm sorry . . .'

Talk about cringing. She did come and sort us out. She could tell I was sorry. What would I ever do without her?

22nd November 2008

We're doing the *OK!* shoot today. The best thing about doing these is getting gorgeous pictures of me and my boys. The crew were really nice. We did loads of shots in the house, messing about in bed and baking things with flour.

The boys got to jump on the bed, which they loved. It's quite hard work for them, smiling and pretending the whole time, but they do a great job.

I had to bribe them by saying they could keep the Scalextric the photo people had brought along with them.

The boys loved the messy bits—chucking flour at me was a dream come true for them. Batman, our Dachshund, got absolutely covered in it and looked like one of those albino dogs.

It took me ages to clean up afterwards. You'd think *OK!* would have sent some cleaners as part of the deal!

I know people say I am doing this for the

money—and yeah, of course I am.

It's not for a flash car or a bigger house now. It's for my kids' bank accounts, just in case I am not around.

I hate thinking like this, but if I wasn't famous and the magazines weren't interested I'd feel even worse.

It makes me feel better knowing I am doing this. There is one thing for certain—my boys won't have the same miserable, poverty-stricken childhood I did.

I was invited back to appear at the reunion of *Bigg Boss* today but there was no way I could go because I am too ill to fly. I wish them all the best, though. It was a lovely bunch of people in there and it was nice of them to ask me.

Went out with the girls—Caroline, Kel and Jen—to Mojos in South Woodford. I just rang them up and said 'I want to go out dancing!' Of course they were well up for it.

I wore thick tights, flat shoes and a woolly cardigan because I've started to feel the cold a lot recently. I felt a bit guilty clubbing when Jack is in prison, but I so badly wanted to have fun.

Caroline said I looked like a prisoner who'd escaped after ten years inside. I just wanted to let my hair down—and we did.

23rd November 2008

I keep thinking about what will happen to my boys if I am not here any more.

Yes, they would go and live with Jeff—but even thinking about it tears me apart.

Not because he can't do it, but because my kids are only little and they need their mum.

Whatever else I may be, I know I'm a bloody good mum. I am their rock. They only go and see their dad every other weekend.

I teach them manners, take them to football, tell them off if they're naughty, and read their bedtime stories. There is no one else who can do it like I can.

I worry if I'm not here to do it, will it be done properly? Will they have the right school uniform and eat up their dinners?

Oh god—what if the worst happens and they forget me? Freddy is only four, so he won't remember much. Bobby is a bit more grown-up and realises more is wrong. I keep thinking back to what I remember from that age, and it's not much.

What if they never know just how much I love them, how very proud of them I am? They are the best thing I have ever achieved and I might not be here to tell them that.

It's like a whole new world of pain whenever I think about it.

So I must stop thinking about it.

I just have to make sure I live.

24th November 2008

Did Christmas dinner for the girls tonight as I'm supposed to be starting chemo again on the 1st of December and I might not have the energy to entertain.

I love my roast dinners—they're wicked. The girls are always surprised at just how good a cook I am. I make lovely lamb shank, shepherd's pie, spag bol, all sorts. I guess I taught myself to cook at a young age as I was left on my own so much.

I had awful stomach cramps when I went to bed after, though. I had to call the doctor at 4am to come out and give me an injection of painkillers and that seemed to do the trick.

25th November 2008

I got Jack's name tattooed in beautiful writing on the inside of my wrist today. My mates were like: 'Jade, that is really sweet but weird for you to put names on your body.'

It didn't half hurt. I stuffed the whole of my jumper in my mouth to stop me from screaming!

I kept having to say 'Sugar' because the cameras were filming and I am not allowed to swear. I would have done if they weren't, believe me. It took longer than I expected and I was shocked at seeing men getting huge tattoos done at the same time. I couldn't understand how they stood the pain.

I love Jack. I can't wait for him to see it as it's my way of showing I care.

He won't be home for Christmas and I can't buy him a present to send so this is the next best thing.

Jen saw it and said: 'But Jade, why has it been written upside down?'

I don't care. It's upside down when I look at my wrist but it will be the right way round when I show to other people.

Funnily enough, my mum once got a tattoo of my dad's name done on her arm. The only trouble was that he'd told her his name was Cyrus when it was actually Andrew.

I know tattoos are permanent but if it all goes tits up I can always add an 'iey' for my mum. Not that I think it will.

Jack and I have talked over the phone about getting married. He says he wants to when he gets out. I feel the same. I know we've been on and off more times than a cop-car light, but we'll make it in the end.

'I love you and always have and always will,' he tells me on the phone.

I want two weddings—one abroad, somewhere hot with close family and friends and then another at home with a big party.

I'm so happy that he has finally said he wants to do it. I'm more in love with him than ever.

Mark rang, he's still trying to talk me out of doing the panto in December but I'm having none of it. Then he told me that Jeff has had a chat with a magazine. Apparently, he was mouthing off about money and who pays for what. He is a good dad but sometimes it feels as if I pay for everything. Move on, Jeff!

I tried to cut the grass to work out my bad mood but the lawnmower was broken!

26th November 2008

I saw in the papers today that Trisha Goddard has beaten breast cancer. Well done, babe!

I also read she's been running every day during the treatment. That's amazing. I would love to be able to do that but what with my hysterectomy and

101

going through the menopause, I just feel totally knackered walking up the stairs these days.

Good on you, Trisha. You're an inspiration. Surely if she can make it then I can as well because I'm younger than her (I think).

There are some nasty people still trying to make out I'm not that ill because I'm still photographed doing the shopping and taking the boys out, and this makes me so upset. I'm a mother to those boys! Of course I'm still looking after them. Mark suggests I mention in my column in *New* that Trisha ran every day during her treatment. I'm not the only one who tries to keep things as normal as possible.

Jen says it's funny how when she reads my column I mention celebrities like Trisha but I never talk about them to my friends. We just talk about normal everyday things like our relationships and our kids (for those who have them) and clothes and so on.

I suppose I have my famous world and my normal world and the two don't mix. That's the way I like it. It keeps things real.

27th November 2008

Went to Winter Wonderland in Hyde Park with the boys. I wanted to take them to Lapland but it couldn't be arranged in time. Danny and Simon know the guys who do this event in Hyde Park so they sorted us some tickets.

It was such a laugh sliding down the slides, eating toffee apples, going on rides and all that.

There was an ice rink so we went skating too.

Poor Freddy was terrified, but I'm pretty good! I was going backwards and everything. They should get me on *Dancing on Ice*.

We went on a rollercoaster too. The film crew came with us and none of us had realised just how fast and scary it was. Poor Bobby screamed his head off and Freddy went quiet with shock.

I wasn't half scared as well.

We went to visit Father Christmas afterwards. Freddy and Bobby asked him how he gets into the houses that don't have chimneys. When he told them he slips through the cracks, my children were like: 'He's not the real one, Mum. The real one uses magic dust!'

I felt so happy the boys had their mum back. I don't feel too bad energy-wise. Bit knackered by the end of the day. It is just so nice to spend a bit of quality time with them. I haven't had any treatment for a couple of weeks now and feel okay.

Alex Curran sent me a message of support. Jonathan Ross also sent me flowers. It's nice they're thinking about me.

28th November 2008

Did a photo shoot and interview today for *New* magazine, who run my column. I felt like crap in the morning with awful niggling pains in my sides. I sat in the car on the way there, clutching my side in pain.

'Let's go home,' Mark said. 'You really don't look well.'

'I'll be fine,' I kept saying, wishing I'd taken painkillers before we left.

We arrived at the studio in east London and it was freezing but I soon started smiling when I saw my costume. I had to play a 1950s housewife, a role I slipped right into. At first when I saw the blonde wig and the 50s dress I thought it looked cheesy, but I have to say it did look good on camera.

Kate said being blonde suits me and I should get a blonde wig when I lose my hair.

Was she joking? People said I looked like Miss Piggy with blonde hair. When I first came out of the *Big Brother* house people were even holding up signs saying 'Kill the pig'! I guess that tight pink dress I was wearing didn't help!

I wouldn't like to go back to those days! I've been brunette ever since, I think.

Maybe it's because of my personality that people think I suit blonde—you know, dizzy blonde and all that! Just goes to show you don't have to be serious if you're dark-haired, though.

After the photo shoot it was on to a video shoot in Stratford with a new singer called Omar Simon.

All the video people said I was a great actress. I had to do a scene where I looked sad through some rainy windows and I got right into it. I really liked the new track and had a little dance with Omar.

It's true what they say that laughter is the best medicine sometimes.

'Right,' I said to Mark. 'I want to go to Hollywood. This is what I should be doing.'

Whack! I turned round at that point and bumped heads with someone! As usual I got carried away, even though Mark was worried and hassling me to leave.

I was knackered.

It was a manic day but I knew it would cheer me up and it did.

All the pain seemed to melt away when the cameras started rolling.

29th November 2008

Felt so ill. The filming had wiped me out so I spent the morning in bed after caring for the boys.

Then Caroline rang me up and asked me out to lunch, so I decided to make the effort. We had a girly chat and she told me about her new bloke, who sounds nice.

We went shopping after and I spent £600 on shoes and clothes. I love splashing out every now and then.

Then I dyed my hair ginger with a packet from Superdrug—which I thought looked great—and met Jen and her boyfriend Mark in the pub.

Our little dachshund Batman is doing my head in. He was a present from Jack to the boys and me last February and when we first had him he was only a puppy. When they're little you put up with the odd accident. But he's not a pup any more and still refuses to go to the toilet outside so I'm always having to mop up after him. Something has to be done—but what?

Some of the papers are saying you shouldn't have tattoos done if you're having chemo. They say there is a high risk of infection. Well, my doctors said it wasn't a problem. Why is everyone on my case all the time? Can't have a massage, can't have a booze-up, can't have tattoos, can't go

105

on sunbeds, can't even have hot baths. What will they try to ban next?

30th November 2008

Went to a pub for my friend Angie's leaving do. She is going travelling and I am so jealous of her! Wish I was going. I'd love to take the boys away too, to show them the world, see the sights and all that.

After all this crap—cancer, Jack in prison, and everything—I fancy moving to Australia and getting a normal job, like being a beautician. Or retraining as a dental nurse, which is what I was doing before *BB3*. I could take my qualifications again over there if I need to. No one would know who I was. I'd never get any grief.

I want to walk the boys to school in flip-flops and go on the beach and breathe fresh air. Have a normal life.

I think Jack would be up for it too. I bet he'd like to get away from all the problems we've had here. I'll ask him later . . .

It's nice to remember that the world is big enough and you can always find somewhere to get away. It would have to be somewhere they speak English, though, because I have enough trouble with the language I know without trying to learn a new one!

Chapter Ten

Getting Ready for Christmas

3rd December 2008

Bobby and Freddy were making Christmas cards today, getting glue and glitter stuck everywhere. I don't mind a bit of glitter, though.

They are getting so excited about Christmas. Now they are at an age where they can understand everything it's lovely.

I go to town with all the Santa Claus stuff. It should be the law that all little kids believe in him. He is real anyway, isn't he?

I am missing a chemo appointment tomorrow. I didn't get a phone call when I expected to get one so I missed the blood test you are supposed to have before the session. I wanted to change the date and couldn't do the next one.

I mentioned it to Kate.

'You're not trying to avoid it, are you?' she asked.

Maybe there was an element of that. I dread the chemo because it makes me feel so shit. This time I knew what I was in for so maybe I forgot it accidentally on purpose.

You just have to be so organised and I am not good at keeping up with this. I am doing my best. I go to almost all of my appointments and any I miss, the hospital reschedule.

I know I need this treatment. It's saving my life.

I nipped over to see Jack's family today. His little brother Louis was looking at some funny bald pictures on the internet.

'That's what you'll look like soon,' he said, taking the mick. He cracked me up.

He's right, though. The nurses told me I'll lose my hair at the beginning of January. It's incredible what these medical people can predict.

The chemo has been rescheduled for the 15th and I'm relieved it's not today. I'm really dreading this next, stronger stuff they're going to fill me up with.

Met the Living crew to drive into town. On the way they picked up some sandwiches from a shop. I went with them because they never get enough food.

We bought those pepperami things as well. After eating loads, Kate and I kept making each other laugh. We felt so sick! Then Kate looked at the wrapper of the pepperami and noticed it was out of date so we felt even sicker!

In the end we had to pull the car over on Tower Bridge Road and I threw up, but it still didn't stop us from laughing. Some men in suits looked at us like we were off our heads.

When we arrived at Max Clifford's office I told Kate to look professional because it's a serious place. She kept on laughing though.

'Look at you, a professional TV person who can't stop cracking up!' I teased her.

In the waiting room she asked me to try and get my leg over my head. I nearly managed it too.

The meeting with Max and Mark today was to talk about work. I gave them both their Christmas presents—a bag of Mulberry bathroom stuff for each of them and a gift for Lucy, who's head of PR at Max's office—and we had a chat about things. Max is a very busy man but he always takes the time if I pop in.

Max said whatever happens my health has to come first, but as long as I feel okay I can carry on. It's up to me.

To be honest I've not looked up any stuff about my cancer. I don't want to know.

I don't know where this has come from, or why certain people get cancer and not others.

I just look at it as something that needs sorting. I might be naïve but I'll take my medication and look forward to getting better.

At the end of the day I am just a single mum who isn't that bright. I'll let the doctors worry about what to do and I'll follow their orders (not like me to follow orders, but no choice really).

I wrapped up a few presents tonight on camera for the Living girls, and ended up chipping my teeth on sellotape. I never knew it was that dangerous!

Even though I am having a break from treatment, I'm getting a few bald patches on my head now. I texted my friend Jen to tell her.

'Are you sure, Jade?' she wrote back.

She knows I exaggerate things sometimes. This time I'm sure, though.

'100 per cent,' I said. 'I just wanted you to know to prepare you.'

I am trying to take this in my stride. There are plenty of people in the same boat as me or who go bald with alopecia. I keep telling myself that life and health are more important than hair. This is not the worst part of having cancer. Not by a long way.

5th December 2008

I went on *This Morning* with Philip and Fern to promote my show.

We were running late and I had to get out of the car, take my coat off, get my nose powdered and walk straight onto the set. There was no time to work out what to say, but I never need help! I don't get nervous either. It just doesn't bother me.

They asked me why I was doing the panto in Lincoln and looked at me like I should be in bed. That's not me though.

Philip said: 'You've got a really intensive period of treatment starting soon and panto two days later. Is that wise?'

I explained to him that people deal with illness in different ways and while I can still work I will. As long as I can get up and walk about I am going to carry on. Why not?

Plus, being honest, I do need the money. I have a mortgage to pay and my boys' school fees and everything. Rightly or wrongly, my living expenses are £11K a month. I know that's loads but when you earn more you spend more, simple as. So unless we move house or change schools I have to keep that up.

Plus there are only so many manicures you can have and shops you can visit. I am not a lady of leisure by nature! I'm glad I'm not just sitting at home thinking: 'Oh my god I've got cancer, I've got cancer . . .' That would only make me feel even worse. Not that I blame anyone who does. People deal with things in their own different ways.

Afterwards I had lots of TV and magazine interviews to do and I kept looking at my watch as Bobby's school play was at 4pm. It's a nativity play in the local church and he is singing in a choir. There was no way I was missing that!

All the interviews were about me working and how I feel etc. One journalist got all narky, asking: 'Do you really think you should be working?' I got pissed off, looked her in the eye, and asked if she had any kids?

'I earn money for my children. Do you have an issue with that?'

She looked a bit guilty and to be honest I hope she felt it. I am just trying to do my best for them. Surely no one can knock me for that?

Finally we left and raced to the school. The driver got lost on the way and I had to ring Kate to get us back on track. Only just made it in time, thank God. Jeff turned up too. Bobby gave us the thumbs-up. Mum had been there keeping him calm, promising him we'd make it. And he was fantastic—a real natural on stage. Afterwards I gave him a big hug and told him how proud I was. Bobby is such a little star.

*　　　*　　　*

Went to the cinema to watch *Four Christmases* with Caroline. She got up to go to the loo after it started so I hid from her when she came back! She got really confused and thought she'd walked into

111

the wrong cinema. It made me laugh so much.

7th December 2008

I went to a book signing at Lakeside shopping centre in Essex. I was supposed to launch the book—*Catch a Falling Star*—a few months ago but it was put back when I got ill.

It goes into detail about my problems in *Celebrity Big Brother* and how I got depressed after all that. I even went into the Priory at one point—what a celeb thing to do! My mum, Kel and Jen all came to see me there. You really find out who your friends are during those dark times.

Anyway, I ended up having a bit of therapy about my anger problems. The whole episode was a proper rock-bottom place. Then just when things were getting better again I got cancer . . . You never know what's round the corner, good or bad.

All the way to Lakeside I was thinking: 'What if no-one comes?' I was worried the event hadn't been advertised very much and I'd be standing on my own feeling like a right lemon.

But when I arrived there was loads of press and the queue waiting for me to sign was almost out of the shop. Thank God for that!

People were so sweet. Lots of them wanted a picture with me or to stop and chat. Everyone was asking about my health and saying nice things.

One guy kept shouting: 'You're an inspiration, Jade!'

It's funny because I don't look ill or feel that bad at the moment. One little girl showed up with a bald head and I had a chat with her, telling her that would be me soon.

People from the shop next door gave me some Ugg boots and trainers for the boys. They are so lucky!

*   *   *

I found out today that the NHS is offering a cervical cancer vaccine to protect seventeen- and eighteen-year-old girls against the HPV virus. HPV is a sexually-transmitted virus that can lead to cervical cancer, but you don't have to sleep around to get it. I've only slept with eight men in my life and I still got it.

I wish I could go back in time and I would definitely have that vaccine myself.

I want to shout to all the girls in the world to go and get it.

If it saves just one person's life it's worth it.

*   *   *

I had a surprise when I got home. There were some four-legged visitors in the fields behind my house—some beautiful Shetland ponies! I've no idea where they'd come from. The boys were so excited. Bobby said they must be girl ones because they didn't have any willies. I didn't have any food for them so tried giving them some blueberries I had in the fridge.

I called the RSPA—RSPE—RSPCC or whatever the people are who save animals because they look a bit neglected. I just hope no one thinks I nicked them!

I rang my friends to tell them and they thought

113

it was a wind-up.

They are doing me a favour because they are eating my grass and it needed cutting.

Then Mum said the manure was good for the garden so we should keep them.

'You can sort that out for my flowerbeds,' I said.

'Oh, I've got to shovel the shit, have I?' she said. No comment.

Rehearsals start for the panto tomorrow but it's Freddy's first big school play so I will go and see that first.

My commitments to my kids come before anything.

8th December 2008

Freddy looked gorgeous as he played Prince Charming in his play. He's perfect for the role because he is such a charmer. I love sitting among the other parents, looking on proudly, doing normal things.

When I see my little boy up there, I know I've done something right in my life.

His face lit up when he saw me and he waved. Jeff came too, which was good.

Whatever else I do, I know I do my best for them. They go to an amazing private school and can probably already read and do sums better than I can. Giving them the chances I never had is so important to me.

Facing something like cancer brings home so much what they mean to me. I need to be here to watch their achievements. I need to stick around to see what they turn out like.

Afterwards I didn't realise the time and had to rush off to drive to Lincoln for my panto rehearsal to get into my role as the evil Queen Tabloid. I always get cast as the evil Queen for some reason.

It took ages to drive up there and when I arrived, knackered, I had missed the rehearsal. Ooops! Hope they don't think I'm a diva or anything. I don't actually know my lines either! I'll make it up to them in the morning. I always fluff things till the last minute but you can rely on Jade on the night!

They booked me into an apartment to stay. It was okay, but I was gutted there wasn't a bath. I so badly need baths. I rang Mark in tears. 'I don't want them to think I'm difficult but I really need a bath. Cool water is the only thing that works on my aching bones.'

He said I should check into a nearby hotel and not to worry.

So I did. I need a bath for the boys as well in case they come up and visit. I can't say I'm looking forward to being away from them again.

9th December 2008

Had the first rehearsals today and I am absolutely shattered.

The cast are all lovely. They don't treat me any differently to anyone else, which I love. I know people look at me and think 'Wow, she has cancer', but hopefully I am showing them it doesn't have to mean the end.

If I am tired, I sit down. If I need to take my pills, I just take them. It doesn't have to be some big drama.

It is tiring, though. I rehearsed for hours, singing and doing my dancing parts. Still, I'd much rather be belting out songs and learning lines than having chemo. Only six more days before that starts again.

The director Chris Colby said I am a natural and look as though I've been in theatre since the age of three. He says he doesn't know where I get it from.

All I can say is, growing up in my house I had to learn how to act. When my mum had drug dealers at the door, I'd say she was out. Or when she was down and needed looking after I'd try and make her laugh.

I hated my friends knowing my dad was a junkie, so I pretended to all of them that Mum was a saint when really she wasn't. Looking back I've been acting all my life. I got an A for GCSE drama and that was the only decent mark I ever got at school.

Kevin Kennedy, who played Curly in *Corrie*, was also starring in it. He was so lovely and said on camera that I was an inspiration for doing it while being ill.

I had a singing rehearsal this morning and a dance one in the afternoon. The singing went well. Back in 2006 I won *Celebrity Stars in your Eyes* playing Lynn Anderson singing 'I Never Promised You a Rose Garden'. I looked a right state wearing that long blonde wig and people obviously thought 'What's she doing up there?', but my voice proved

116

them wrong. I can belt them out when I get going, even if I sometimes forget the words.

The musical director kept telling me not to smile and to act more evil, so I really went for it. Luckily this treatment hasn't affected my voice. I am still the loudest person in there.

Then I had to go for a dance lesson at the Lincoln Labour Club across town.

It was freezing in there. I gave it my all but it took its toll.

I've got a bag full of loads of pills to take when I'm in pain. I'm not bad at swallowing them, but some are bigger than others and make me want to gag.

Got back totally exhausted. The panto people have found a house with a bath in it for me—what a relief!

14th December 2008

Today I visited Jack in Wayland Prison, Norfolk, and he gave me a rose that he'd saved up for with his convict's money.

I looked round and saw other prisoners holding two or three roses for their partners.

'How come I'm only getting one?' I laughed.

'I knew you'd say that,' said Jack. 'It's just they get more money for their jobs than me.'

It was so lovely to see him. I can't wait until he comes out. We talked a bit about the treatment and our plans for the future.

Jack says he saw a programme about the Seven Wonders of the World on TV and it stuck in his head.

'I want to take you to them all and then propose when we get to the last one,' he said.

I smiled, then frowned. 'You shouldn't have told me about it because it won't be a surprise any more.'

I am glad he has been thinking about proposing, though. It makes me feel all fuzzy and warm inside.

Chapter Eleven

The Show Must Go On

15th December 2008

They're having a technical rehearsal for the panto today but my rearranged chemotherapy is starting again so I have to go to the Marsden in the morning.

They put a new line into my heart area first of all. It makes me cry every single time. What a horrible thing to have done.

I felt so impatient as I waited for all the bags of saline to wash me out.

'Let me go,' I said to the nurses. 'I'll just drink more or something!'

But they've got their routines and you just have to go along with it.

I do have good news, though, Dr Ind tells me the cancer cells have shrunk a little, so that means the chemo is working. Yippeeee!!!

Afterwards I got straight back into the car and drove to Lincoln. The panto opens in two days and I still don't know my lines. I just sing: 'La la la

118

laaaaa' when I forget my songs.

I had a bit of a practice with the Living TV crew sitting in the car park at lunchtime to try and get my head round the words.

I'm sure I'll pull it out the bag in time. I almost always do.

16th December 2008

Dress rehearsal today. My new tablets are making me jittery and I talk at hundreds of miles an hour. Kate could hardly understand a word I was saying. And I was sick in the theatre car park when we arrived. My tummy is all over the place again.

Looking back, I've had problems with going to the toilet for years now. Last summer, I went away with Danielle to a caravan park and ended up constipated and even blew off on camera while they were filming the Living show I was doing back then! It cracked me up! I had back pains too, but never ever thought it was anything as serious as this. I had cancer then and no clue.

I'm glad I have the Living crew with me. We spend the evenings together and they are good mates to have around.

Actually I love my whole team at the moment— my agent Mark, my friends, and my mum is being brilliant. There are lots of good people around me. If anything gets me through this, they will.

In my head I think to myself I have to get better, but in my heart, if I am being honest, I just don't know. In a way that makes it more important than ever to work for money. I need it for the boys.

17th December 2008

Mum brought the boys along for my first night. We had one early performance for the kids and then the evening do.

I loved getting dressed up and hoped I'd make my boys and Mum proud of me. Hope they are not scared of me either! I do try my best to be evil.

Before it we had had another quick run-through and that had already knackered me. I had to rise up through a trap door with freezing smoky ice stuff around me at one point and I just kept wobbling and felt as though I was about to fall over.

I got a strange present in the dressing room just before I went on. Someone called Ivor had sent me dozens of beautiful roses and a sparkly ring. He said I was gorgeous! No clue who he is. Hope Jack doesn't get jealous.

When I got on stage everyone started cheering straight away. What a buzz! But that wasn't right because I am supposed to be evil.

'You're supposed to boo!' I shouted at the audience.

I could see my boys in the circle screaming: 'Come on, Mum!'

I loved every minute. I never get nervous because if I forget my lines I just make them up! People don't seem to mind.

Afterwards the tiredness really hit me. My limbs were so heavy and my feet were killing me because of the high shoes have to wear.

By the time I did my bow (where my hat was nearly falling off!) I was desperate to lie down.

I put the boys in their PJs at the hotel and Mum took them home.

Bobby said 'Mummy, you were really good.' That meant more to me than anything a reviewer could ever say. It was the best praise in the world to me.

18th December 2008

I did two shows today but I was so tired I really had to force the smile onto my face when the curtain went up. Once I felt the energy of the crowd I soon got into it.

The papers have been saying nice things about my performance and that I am doing alright. I played the Wicked Queen in a Gravesend panto back in 2002 and it went well then. People think you're on your way out if you're famous and in panto, but actually they are loads of fun and make you feel good.

It's a buzz being on stage and I'd like to do more of it.

*   *   *

Later on, I heard that Katie Price said some kind things in a magazine interview. She said she didn't realise how sick I was and that she now respects the fact I'm still working and providing for my children.

I got choked hearing this. It really does mean a lot to me that people understand why I'm doing this. It's not about me needing the limelight or trying to publicise myself. At this stage, it's all for

Bobby and Freddy.

I realise now what a waste of energy it is being angry with people. I'm glad Katie said sorry. I want to make peace with everyone.

19th December 2008

After the show, my tummy felt so poorly all I wanted to do was lie down. Then I started to be sick, over and over in the loo. I just couldn't stop, even after there was nothing left to come up. It was horrible.

I rang Mark and said: 'Get me out of here!'

'Jade, you're pushing yourself too hard,' he told me. 'You should never have taken this on.'

For once I had to agree with him. He had warned me it would be tough but I ignored him because I so wanted to do it!

I am taking tomorrow morning off. I just need my bed.

20th December 2008

My stand-in had to do the afternoon performance today but I managed to go back on stage for the evening.

When I spoke to Jack, he told me off. 'You should be taking it easy and stop rushing around doing all this.'

'I can't,' I replied. 'I want a normal life.' Whatever normal means.

I don't want to let people down. If they have booked tickets to come and see the show because I am on the poster, then they should be able to see me on stage when they turn up. At the end of the day I like working and agreed to do this. A lot of effort goes into a show like this. I just have to pick myself up and carry on.

21st December 2008

I did two shows today and got really, really tired. In between, I kept necking my pills. If I move too quickly I'm gonna start rattling!

It's hard keeping up with what I need to take and when but I think I am taking them at the right times. Kate helps me sometimes. I decided to stay in the crew's hotel because it's nice to have someone to chat to of an evening and get that bit of extra support.

22nd December 2008

I did my afternoon show at the panto and then went home to Essex, so tired I could hardly walk. I wanted to go to bed but I had a dog trainer coming round to help me with Batman.

I was at my wit's end after Mum told me he'd peed on the white leather sofa. The trainer says I should stop telling him off and get him into a routine of going outside to the toilet. I am not convinced he understands what we want him to do, though. That dog has a mind of his own.

As a joke, I told Freddy I was going to send him to a sausage factory. Well, I thought it was funny at least.

Exhausted is not the word. I can hardly get up and down the stairs. This is not funny.

As much as I love the boys I am struggling a bit to keep up with them. Both are little whirlwinds, especially Bobby.

There was no way I could do the evening show tonight but when they heard they were very understanding about it, thank God! It's been agreed I'll have a break till after Christmas.

23rd December 2008

A strange woman turned up at the door today wearing huge hoop earrings and a tracksuit. She reminded me of Vicky Pollard.

'Hello, I've come to see you. Your mum said I could,' she told me.

I didn't know her from Adam but I don't like to offend people so I said she could come in. She looked well chuffed.

I called to Mum and asked her: 'Do you know who this lady is?'

She just shrugged! She had no idea.

Then I realised I'd invited a total stranger into my house. She started telling me she was staying for dinner, then she went into my living room and I heard her ring up her mate and say: 'You'll never guess where I am? Jade Goody's house!'

To wind me up, Mum invited her to stay for dinner. I can't believe she did that! Luckily the lady seemed pleased enough just to wander round for a bit and then leave.

How strange was that?

Tonight I went out to a party for Steve Jones, who worked with me on *Jade's Salon*.

I decided to wear a headscarf because the bald patches on my head look horrible. People were lovely about it.

We had a laugh and a bit of a dance then I whacked my head on a cupboard in the bar and felt as though I had a dent in it! I took my headscarf off to check then I just thought sod it and left it off.

Of course, someone tried to take my picture and I decided we had to leave. I had to get home anyway to take a tablet. My life revolves around taking pills now. I got annoyed with Mum because she was trying to chat up some girl (she's gay, in case anyone out there hadn't realised) and she was keeping me waiting. When I need to go, I need to go straight away.

Christmas Eve, 2008

I'm all snotty and seem to have caught a cold. I was so tired too, until the excitement of preparing for Christmas took over! I turn into a big kid myself. I love it.

Bobby and Freddy wrote their letters to Santa and we burned them on the fire. Oh, I love having a proper fire! Makes me feel all Christmassy!

I told them: 'After it goes up the chimney the pieces of letters all stick together again so Santa can read them.'

They seemed to believe me. I love the look on their little faces.

Note: my boys are not allowed to read the above until they are at least twelve. I want them to believe in Santa for as long as possible. It's so magical.

I wanted to organise fake snow for the garden so the boys could leap out of bed and get a surprise on Christmas morning, but it's too late to arrange now.

Instead, I threw some talc on the living-room floor and stamped fake Santa boots in it. I bit into the carrot the boys had left out and poured their glass of milk down the sink.

Mum and I stayed up in our PJs to wrap up a few last-minute presents. I'd bought a massive dinosaur for the boys but couldn't get the damn thing put together. It was so complicated. Someone can do it for me tomorrow.

I never had many Christmas presents when I was growing up. We were so hard-up. One year the electricity ran out and we had to light the room with candles. Which was fine until the room caught fire and nearly burned our council house down.

I feel so much closer to Mum these days—just like I did when I was really little, before all the drug stuff happened.

We still argue but now we make it up fast. We send each other text messages saying 'sorry' after falling out instead of leaving it weeks before we speak again.

People always say things happen for a reason and I like to think my cancer will bring me closer to her for good.

When I am better our relationship will be much stronger and we can thank my cancer for that.

I had to keep going upstairs to check on Bobby and Freddy. They were too excited to drop off to sleep tonight. It's hard because I could easily go to bed earlier than them these days. Come seven o'clock I'm running out of juice, big time.

Christmas Day, 2008

The boys woke up so early, desperate to open their presents. I spoilt them a bit this year, I must admit. They got games, toys and Santa got them quad bikes as well. We couldn't get them started to begin with until Char's bloke realised they needed petrol to work. I must admit they went a bit faster than I realised and I felt nervous. They looked so small underneath the big helmets! They absolutely loved them though and were soon tearing round the garden.

My mum bought me underwear, PJs and a lovely jumper. I got sent some Jo Malone bath oil and four fab pairs of Love from Australia boots too.

My nan and granddad bought me a massive jumper. I think it will look alright if I take the belt off it. I couldn't help laughing at it though (sorry, guys!).

Jack got his mum to buy me a gorgeous bag from Reiss; he knows how much I love the stuff from there.

We managed to have a quick chat on the phone. He told me he got a tin of cranberry sauce from his cellmate. He's been getting his mum to copy CDs onto cassette for inmates who don't have much. He's so sweet.

I bought him a jumper and trousers from All Saints, which I knew he'd love.

It was good to hear his voice but he was gutted to miss Christmas. Every year he's always got right into it with the boys. Last year he filled the room with hundreds of balloons he blew up himself and he covered my house in every kind of Christmas decoration. He's like a big kid and no one loves this time of year more than him.

But Christmas in prison is like any other day in prison.

'When I get out we'll have our own special Christmas later on in the year,' he said. 'We'll do it properly with the works.'

*   *   *

Thankfully I was well enough to have everyone round and I cooked the dinner myself. I really went to town with the food, making turkey, duck and lamb as well so everyone could choose what they wanted. I do love cooking my Christmas dinners. There were thirteen of us today—Mum, Nan, Grandad, Charlene and her boyfriend, the boys and me, and the Living TV crew who were filming us.

I did far too much food as usual and gave my grandparents some to go home with. (They were a bit merry as usual!)

The boys went off to Jeff's in the evening. I'd packed Mum off too as she needed a break from it all, and when everyone left I watched an old movie and had a bit of a cry. I was starting to feel ill again and just felt really lonely.

I'm so tired I can barely manage the stairs.

Boxing Day, 2008

Woke up feeling so terrible I didn't know what to do. I ran into the bathroom and retched in the toilet bowl. I am getting good at this.

Called the doctor and he reckons it's the norovirus—that vomiting bug.

'What?' I said. 'I can't be unlucky enough to get that on top of cancer, can I?'

There should be a rule that if you have cancer you don't get anything else.

The doctor said my immune system is very low now so I should try and stay indoors and not use anyone else's toilets in case I catch anything.

There was no way I could make it to the panto and I felt terrible for all those people who'd bought tickets to see me. The boys were at their dad's too and that always makes me feel worse. They give me a reason to perk up. The house was so empty and I just felt so low.

It was hitting me hard about Jack not being here either. *Why isn't he here when I need him the most?*

Ended up just going to bed early and trying to sleep off this mood.

27th December 2008

I didn't feel any better when I woke up and I knew there was no way I could do the panto later. Mark rang to explain to them. It made me feel even more depressed that I was letting everyone down.

I'm glad in a way that Christmas is over for

another year. I hope next year's is much happier for all of us. *I hope I'm cured by then. I must be.*

I felt like crap all day and by the evening I was so lonely that I rang Jen and her sister Angela to go out for a drink. I knew it was a stupid idea but I needed to do something or I would have gone mental.

'Come on then,' Jen said. 'I could do with cheering up.' She was feeling rubbish too as her boyfriend had just dumped her—at Christmas! What a dickhead.

I'm not meant to drink but we went to Faces in Essex and I picked up a few bottles of champagne to share. One or two glasses won't hurt, I'm sure.

When I got to the bar to pay I went to put my PIN number in and I'd forgotten what it was! It's on my mobile, which was in my car, so I had to rush outside and get it then call Angela over the phone from the car park and tell her what it was. She kept asking me to repeat it, we were giggling so much.

Mum found out I was out drinking and she rang Jen and had a go at her. I only had one mum—honest! I know she worries so much about me now. It's funny because in the past, I would have been the one telling her off!

We had a bit of a dance and I just let my hair down for a change. I know it was mad. I know I shouldn't have gone out at all, but I needed to pick myself up and at least it did the trick.

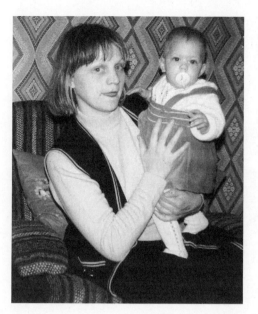

Mum was so proud of me. I probably needed the dummy though—the only time she got any peace!

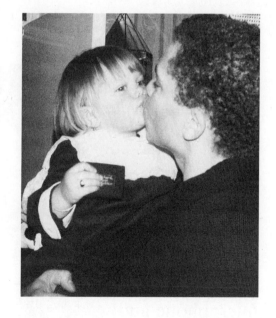

A kiss for Daddy's Princess. I know he loved me really. Just a shame he wasn't around to prove it.

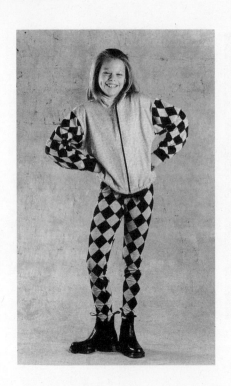

Check out those chequered patterns! This was from a promo shot for my modelling.

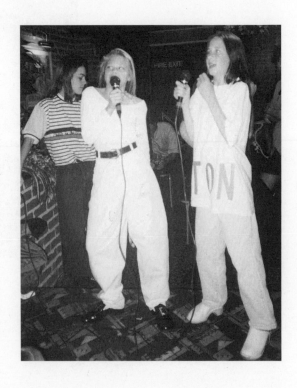

Ha ha! The good old days of white baggy jeans. If there's a microphone and music on I can't stop myself.

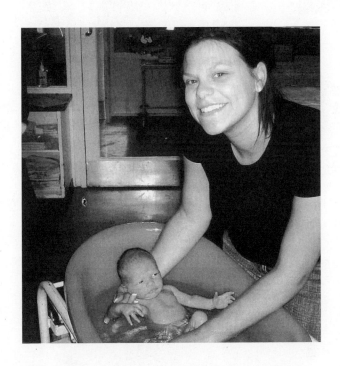

Freddy's first bath. I was facing life as a single mum, but I told myself: 'Just get on with it!'

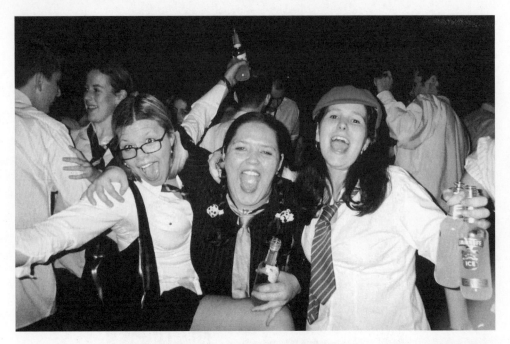

Watch out, us girls are about! One of many we would have that night.

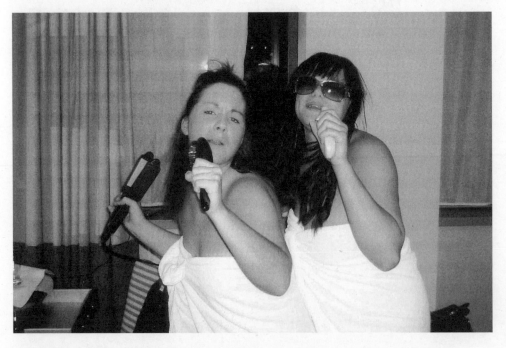

A spot of hairbrush singing to get us in the mood for another big night out.

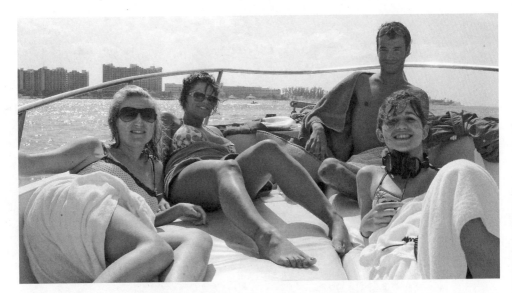

Boat trip with Jack and our mates in the Bahamas, 2006.
We had some wicked times in the sun.

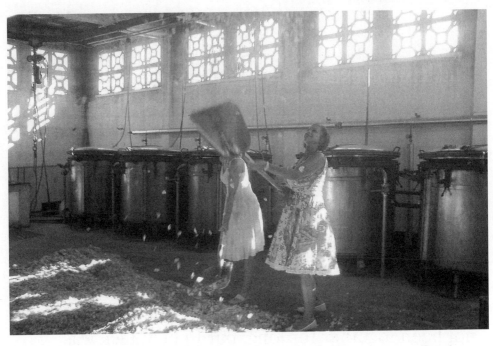

I absolutely loved doing the research for my perfumes.
I was really hands on and proud of the scent I chose.

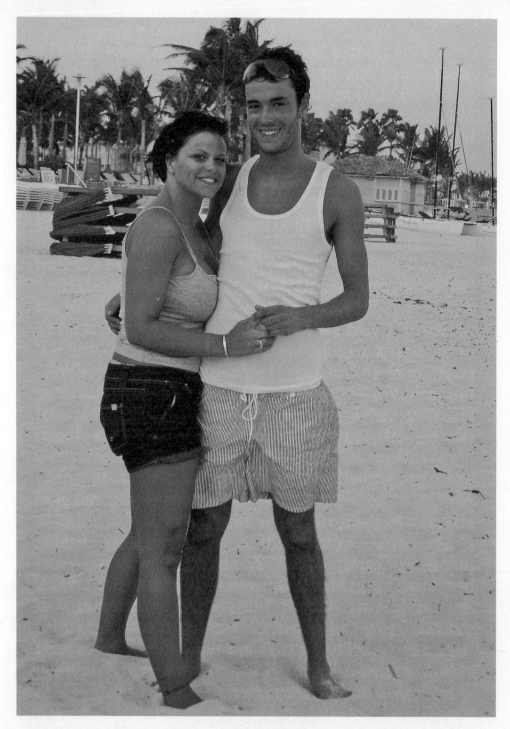

Me and my boy on the beach, Bahamas, 2006. We'd not been together for long, but I knew Jack was special.

28th December 2008

Mark and I had a chat and decided I have to pull out of the panto. I'm just not well enough. He says he will explain it to them. I feel really bad about it but at least my stand-in will get a chance at it now. It will be good news for someone!

I felt okay today, then the pain started again and got worse and worse.

'I was alright earlier,' I cried to Jack. 'What's going on inside my body?'

'Jade, you have to calm down and take it easier,' he said.

Everyone's telling me that. I think I might have to start listening.

31st December 2008

Last night I was in horrible pain and went back to the Marsden.

The doctors gave me a scan and decided my kidneys have got blocked and I will need emergency surgery. *Great. Yet another operation.*

I never know what's going to happen next. It's frightening.

Luckily, they only kept me in for a few hours.

After that the boys and I went round to Kev's house to spend New Year's Eve with his family. We had food and watched Elton John's gig on TV. Kev told me that Elton has offered me his Spanish villa when I need a rest. I might take him up on that!

I told my mum to go out and enjoy herself tonight. She deserves a break and to be honest we need a little rest from each other every now and

then. Even if we sometimes fight over silly things—
it's always the really little things that cause the
biggest fights!—we know we'll make up again
within the hour. She's being amazing to me just
now.

Chaper Twelve

The Bald Truth

1st January 2009

I am wishing so hard that this year will be better
than last! I just keep thinking of all the things I'll
do when I'm better. I keep saying: 'When I'm
better . . . when I'm better . . .'

It's going to include lots of holidays, that's for
sure. I'm still thinking about my Australia idea.
And going to Hollywood!

I know I've been lucky doing this job of being a
reality TV person. I've met amazing people, done
amazing things—like bring out a perfume, make
TV shows, get asked to write books. God I've even
been asked (a couple of years ago) to be in
Playboy! (I decided that the British public had seen
as much of me as they could possibly want when I
stripped off in *BB*!)

But this illness has made me realise that living a
real life is more important. This way of life can't
go on and on forever. It will be time for me to
hang up my boots and move on. I want to be rid of
the stress and the dramas.

And when I get over this hideous disease I

promise myself I'll do that. Just as the anger I had has no place in my life, maybe I need to get a normal job now and settle down with my family.

I am still feeling so ill today. My hair is so thin that I can't even hide the bald patches any more. The nurses are saying it will all have come out by the 8th of January, a week from now, and it looks as though that's going to be true.

2nd January 2009

I woke up this morning to find chunks of hair on my pillow—not just a few hairs but great big lumps of it. I knew it was going to happen. I'd been waiting for it. I'd expected it would happen before and for a few weeks I thought maybe I'd get away with it because my hair's always been quite thick and healthy. Surely I deserve some luck somewhere along the line?

Then I saw it lying next to me when I woke up.

I didn't want to look in the mirror. What a shock! No woman wants to see herself with huge bald patches like that. It had started to go at the front as well so I look like a right slaphead.

As usual I tried to put on a brave face. Mum got a nice silk scarf and tried to show me how to put it on, which is not easy for her with her one working hand.

'Don't look at it, Jade,' she said. 'You don't need to.' I could tell even she was shocked. I am a young woman and I look awful.

That's when the blubbing started. It was like a dam bursting. I sat on my toilet sobbing my heart out.

133

Living TV were filming and I don't usually mind the cameras rolling, but this time I shut the door for a few minutes.

Mum just cradled my balding head tightly while I bawled like a baby.

This was it. I had to face life bald.

I loved her so much at that moment. I've always known she loves me but she was never really good at mothering.

I was only young when she had the accident and lost the use of her arm so I had to do all the chores around the house. I even had to wash her hair when she couldn't manage. I couldn't concentrate at school and kept nodding off in the day because I was having to do all the housework long into the night.

Later on, Mum got into smoking crack with a really dodgy bunch of mates. I knew she was doing it but she wouldn't admit it. After school I'd come home to find her sitting in silence and staring vacantly into the distance. And the house always stank of smoke. I hated her for choosing an evil drug over me at the time, but those days were long ago.

Now, when she held me so close, I was her baby again and she was my mum.

She's giving me strength she never did when I was growing up.

*   *   *

I had to sort myself out as Kev was coming to pick me up and take me to hospital for my kidney operation. They need to sort out the tubes so I can wee properly again. It will only take a couple of

134

hours and they've said I can go home later on.

*   *   *

When I was lying in bed after I came round from the op, I decided to share the news about my hair. I took a simple photo of me looking at the camera with my balding head with just a few wispy strands left then I sent it to everyone on my phone, without a message.

Jen rang me up first. 'Oh my god,' she said. 'Are you okay?'

'Yes,' I said. 'I just wanted you to see it.'

Kate called and said: 'Don't you worry, girl. We'll all wear headscarves too.'

*   *   *

Back at home, the boys came into the living room and caught me crying. I pulled myself together straight away but Bobby burst into tears at the sight of my head.

He said, 'I'm sorry, I don't like it.'

My little boy doesn't want a baldie for a mum!

'Bobby, it's okay,' I tried to soothe him. I told him the story I had decided to tell them about accidentally using hair remover instead of shampoo.

Freddy was great and said: 'Let's all be skinheads! Can I do it too?'

But I am going to keep it covered until they have a chance to come to terms with it. It's not the way you want to see your mummy looking.

3rd January 2009

Even more of my hair has come off now. I look like a newborn baby chick. With my headscarf I feel like a doddering old lady. I like old ladies but never thought I'd look like one at the age of twenty-seven!

I went to Harrods with Mum to buy some lovely new headscarves and I splashed out a bit on four pairs of shoes (I love 'em!) and a make-up bag.

Back home, Mum gave me another lesson in tying my scarves. Kev came round and had a look.

'She's a big black girl now who knows how to do her headscarves,' said Mum.

I rolled my eyes. 'The things you come out with! Just shut your mouth!'

Mum is so tactful—or do I mean '-less'?

7th January 2009

I went to visit Jack for the first time this year. I wore a scarf as I was scared to let him see my bald head. What if he doesn't fancy me any more?

He held my hand and then I let him have a little peek underneath the scarf.

He welled up, right there, sitting in the crowded room.

'It's the first time you've actually looked ill,' he whispered.

He won't talk about the illness on the phone. I say: 'Jack you have to face this,' and he changes the subject.

Then he showed me the new tattoo on his bicep. It reads: 'Live with no regrets.'

Apparently one of the inmates did it with a fork and a needle!

I didn't want to start a row but couldn't help tutting.

'For god's sake, Jack,' I said. 'You could have got an infection.'

He looked a bit embarrassed. 'It absolutely killed,' he said. 'And I don't know why I did it. Think I just got pressured really.'

For a DIY job it does look good, I admit.

I quite like the message. Especially given what we are living through at the moment. I don't want to even think about regrets.

8th January 2009

Another big dose of chemo today. I woke up at 6am and didn't want to get out of bed because my bones felt warm for once. I've been feeling cold a lot since I started this new, more powerful chemo.

Kevin drove me to the hospital and sat with me for the treatment. He doesn't have much fitness work at the moment, he says, so he's happy to come with me. It's really nice of him.

They give you medicine before the chemo and it always makes me feel like stinging nettles are all over my body. I'm itchy as well and sit scratching away.

Afterwards they give you something to make you sleepy.

A nurse told me today that I should shave the rest of my hair off so it grows back all together.

'What is your hair usually like?' she asked.

'Straight and brown,' I said.

'Well, it might grow back curly,' she said.

What the hell am I gonna do with curly hair!?

The crew got permission to film me today and are going to release the pictures but I don't know how interesting they'll be because all I'm doing is lying on a bed. Still, I've never seen anyone having chemo on TV before. I hope it helps some people.

I am not just doing this film for other people but myself too. Once I am better I want to look back and see how bad I was. I knew nothing about cancer before doing this, except that it was a big scary thing that you don't get better from, then you end up brown bread.

There is so much to it. I've learned a lot. I want to look back and feel good about it.

I had a blood transfusion today as well. I've already had four of them. I have never given much thought to giving blood before but it's amazing. Because people are so kind and take the trouble to give it, I can get my energy levels back and feel better sooner.

I don't properly understand how it works, but I know it does. So thank you to everyone who has ever given blood. I might have some of yours!

I wonder if the royal family give it? That could make me blue-blooded now! There's a thought . . .

10th January 2009

The effects of the chemo always seem to kick in on day two or three. I get really tired and run down.

Kate and the Living crew tried to interview me this morning and I just lost it. 'I am not answering any more stupid questions,' I said. 'I am not doing

138

this any more!'

Kate came upstairs with me and I told her I'd had enough. I'm so fed up with all the cancer questions. I seem to talk about it the whole time and I'm bored of hearing my own voice going on about it.

She understood and let me rant and rave. Afterwards I calmed down and changed the subject.

'Let's talk about something fun now!' I said.

I'm going off to Tenerife on holiday in a couple of days and I did a bit of fashion show, showing her all the clothes I've bought for it, including a very fetching black and white swimming cap with flowers on it. That cheered me up.

Looking in the mirror I can see how much weight I've lost. My trousers are hanging off me. I suppose it's one good thing about cancer that it makes you lose loads of weight—but I don't recommend it!

Afterwards the girls—Jen, Kelly and Caroline—came over for the first time since I lost my hair. I always feel like my normal self again when they're around.

Up till now they'd only seen pictures of me looking like a plucked chicken but when they saw the real thing they all said I looked so young. None of them thought they'd be able to pull it off as well as me!

I showed them the Shetland ponies that are still in my garden. I opened the window and shouted at them.

'I pay to live here and you do not and it's my garden so please just leave!'

The girls cracked up.

139

Then we all went to the Piano Lounge in Epping for dinner. I had two starters—a duck salad and prawns—then lamb shank, one of my favourites. I only drank lemonade but told Jen it was wine so she'd get pissed.

'I'm drinking—look,' I said, laughing.

We had a really good chat and at one stage things got a bit emotional. Caroline cried. I know it's hard on all of them. They are all scared for me and finding it hard to take in. I'd feel the same if any of them got cancer. I mean, who gets cancer in their twenties?

We've made a promise to spend one day every month doing something together like a sleep-over, go-karting or wing walking on an aeroplane. Well, not everyone was so enthusiastic about that last one.

I joked that I want to go to a fancy-dress party as a boiled egg. I'd include a spoon hanging out of my head.

It felt so good to see them and do something normal. They've been with me through thick and thin. In a way we're even closer now than ever. My girlfriends are the best!

Chapter Thirteen

Escape to the Sun

11th January 2009

Today we're packing for our holiday. We've been invited to stay with Bob Coleman, the friend who I call my perfume gurry (I'm told the word is actually guru but I prefer my version now). He helped me develop Ssh and Controversial. I was really hands-on choosing the fragrances. Ssshh won awards and everything.

I was the first non-big celebrity to bring out her own perfume. All the others were big stars like Victoria Beckham, Paris Hilton and Beyonce, whereas I'm just a reality TV star with a big gob.

Controversial was brought out as part of my comeback after the *Celebrity BB* thing. I thought it was a bit cheeky calling it that, but people still liked it.

Anyway, we're off to Bob's villa in Tenerife tomorrow and the boys are really excited. I have loads of packing to do. These days I think Bobby and Freddy have almost as many clothes as I do.

12th January 2009

We got up early to go to Gatwick for our flight. My friend Kevin Adams is coming and bringing his daughters so Bobby and Freddy have someone to play with. His wife Helen will be there as well so my mum has someone to get drunk with!

I felt so ill on the way to the airport that I couldn't even walk to the plane. My joints were aching and I had to get a little shuttle bus to the plane with all the old, disabled people.

I was next to one old man who was bald. 'God, it's cold without hair, isn't it?' I said to him, just making conversation.

He looked at me and said, 'I'm sorry you find that.'

Don't think he got the joke!

As usual there was a drama. On the plane the crown on Mum's tooth fell out. She got them done for *Extreme Makeover* in 2006. She had a boob lift, facelift and new teeth, the works. She looked amazing and she was so made up about it she even stopped smoking. My nan and granddad were choked when they saw her. She looked exactly like she had done before her accident all those years ago.

I managed to stick her tooth back in with nail glue, after nearly losing it down the side of the plane seat.

'You'll give me a gum infection,' said Mum.

'Oh, shut up moaning!' I said.

Arriving at Bob and his wife Carole's villa was so good. It's beautiful there and being in the sun felt lovely. They are like a second set of grandparents to me.

I had a chat with Bob by the pool and I could tell from his face how worried he is about me.

My brave face started slipping as we chatted.

He said: 'It doesn't hurt to have a few tears now and then.'

Usually I try never to cry in front of other

people, but I know how much he cares about me so I let it out a bit.

'I'll be okay,' I managed to say.

Please, please, please let me be okay.

13th January 2009

We spent all day long on the beach. I'm keeping my swimming cap on because Mark is negotiating a deal with *News of the World* for them to get exclusive pictures of my bald head and it's worth a lot of money. At the end of the day I'd rather someone takes a nice picture of me, in a photographic studio with good lighting, than someone shoots me with a long lens while I'm putting the rubbish out.

In some ways going public with these big events makes it easier for me to face them.

The boys had a brilliant time in the sand. All kids love the sea. It was so lovely to sit and watch them having fun. We played football and went swimming, all normal fun things.

Oooh and that hot sun on my skin was just what the doctor ordered. Actually they told me to be careful as my skin is more sensitive than usual. A few rays didn't hurt, though.

I have good skin that tans quite easily, probably because of my dad being mixed race.

When I took off my swimming hat I asked my mum and Kev to hold the towel around me as I bent down.

The joker that he is, Kev started thrusting his hips as he stood in front of me, moaning and licking his lips.

'Kev!' I yelled. 'Stop it, you dirty man!'

My mum was cracking up.

She was being a pain about her broken tooth. We were all having hot baguettes on the beach and I got her a soft brown bread roll instead.

'Jade,' she said. 'I don't want no brown horrible bread. I want what you're having.'

'You can't, Mum, 'cos of your tooth. It's too hard.'

Mum being Mum didn't listen, of course. As soon as our backs were turned what did I hear?

'Owwwww!'

She'd only gone and sneaked a bite of baguette and out popped her tooth. Nail glue won't sort it this time. We had to get polygrip.

Later we went out on a boat to see if we could see any of the dolphins that Bob says they sometimes get round there. It got cold and bit choppy so I told them to go back. Then it felt warmer so I asked if they could turn around again. Then it got really choppy so I asked them to turn back but they ignored us this time. I was just a bit nervous being on a rocking boat with my boys. Mum had had a few drinks as well. The captain wasn't sure about letting her on as he didn't want her to be sick on his deck.

We didn't see any dolphins and I was happy to get back on dry land.

In the evening I found some fancy-dress costumes at Bob's house and Carole and I got dressed up and sang Elvis songs. Mum pissed herself laughing (not literally!). It was wicked.

I went to bed but then woke up around 4am to hear the soft footsteps of Mum and Helen trying to slip in unnoticed.

'Mum,' I snapped, feeling like her mother. 'You think I can't hear you—well I can.'

Then I heard Kev saying to Helen: 'What time do you call this?'

Those two are trouble when they pair up!

I am so glad we've got away. I do feel a bit odd, though. I can't quite shake off my cancer because it's always there in my mind. I know what I'm going back home to and wish I could just stay away.

14th January 2009

We went on a trip to a monkey park. Mum managed to kneel in monkey poo and had to use a leaf to wipe it off. Then we went to look at some monkeys that do acrobatics. Mum looked into the cage at one and asked: 'What's he doing?' Then it piddled all over her arm!

Next I made faces at the gorilla and it spat at Mum, who was standing behind me!

'Dirty fucking animals,' she ranted, before storming off.

I was convinced I could talk to them. 'Ooooooh ooooh aaaah aaaaah ahhhhhh.' I'm pretty sure they knew what I was on about.

We saw a parrot that could speak. Trouble was, we said 'Hello' to it so many times it almost lost its voice copying us.

Freddy loves all animals and went mad for it.

And then all too soon it was time to fly home that afternoon. Bob looked really emotional when he said goodbye, which was a bit much for me.

I didn't want him to set me off too.

When we got back, I rang Jack. He'd seen a photo in the papers of me in my swimming hat and says I look like Olive Oil out of Popeye. Thanks, Jack! I'll take that as a compliment, shall I?

15th January 2009

I did an interview with Carole Malone to go with the *News of the World* pictures they're going to run on Sunday. I met Carole in *Celebrity BB* in 2007. She had slagged me off in her columns before, so I was a little bit wary of her. Told her I know she's done at least one column having a go at me but I let it go. Better to get on with her.

We did the photos and I was terrified of taking off my scarf in case everyone said I was an ugly egg, but Carole said I looked really pretty. It was nice of her to say that but I still feel bad that I've lost my femininity. I don't feel sexy any more. Maybe that's trivial when I'm battling to save my life, but I still want to feel like a woman in the middle of all this.

Bobby saw me without my headscarf this morning and he screamed and called me 'Baldie'.

'Don't worry, darling, I'm putting my scarf back on again,' I said.

But how bad is that when your appearance upsets your five-year-old child?

Freddy takes it all in his stride as usual. But I don't.

Carole quizzed me about my boys and having to talk about them was hard.

I told her I never wanted kids before I had them. After growing up in a house with heroin and

146

crack and waiting for the benefits cheque to buy food and clothes only for Mum to spend it on drugs was terrifying. I was scared of taking on that responsibility. Now, of course, my boys are my world. When they were born I realised motherhood is the thing I was born to do. God gave me these boys, this happiness, and I can't let cancer beat it and take it all away.

Then her questioning got tougher and she basically asked me if I have faced the fact that I might not make it. I just started sobbing and told her I have to accept I might not. The words 'I might not make it' and 'I'm terrified what will happen to the boys' are the hardest things of all to say. They send a shiver down my spine.

I told her, 'In my heart I keep telling myself I WILL make it, that I MUST. But in my head, I just dunno.'

I can't bear to think these thoughts. I have to make it. Please, God, help me!

After the shoot Mark and I went for a drink and bumped into a film director I knew from some awards thing, but of course I couldn't remember his name. I nagged Mark to get in touch with him later. Hollywood will be mine!

18th January 2009

My legs were aching so badly when I woke up that I could hardly move. Maybe I've overdone it with everything. I hate not being able to do normal things. It was really scary, like being paralysed. Gradually the feeling returned and I started to feel a bit better.

I picked up a book a friend gave me when I was diagnosed. It's called *Life Application Study Bible*. It helps you to understand how you can live your life following the lessons that are in the bible. I've started taking comfort from some of the things it says and thinking a bit more about religion in general.

*   *   *

The *News of the World* article has come out today. I quite like the pictures. I never thought I'd see a picture of myself on the front of the *NOTW* with a bald head on! But then I never thought I'd get cancer.

It's funny because Bobby seems to accept my baldness a bit more now he's seen me in the paper. He's used to seeing my face splashed everywhere.

I called Charlene. 'Seen the photos?' I asked.

'Yeah,' she replied.

'What do you think?'

'You pull it off, to be fair,' she said.

'You've got to say that because you're my friend,' I laughed.

Mary said I looked so stunning. 'You could even get married looking like that, Jade,' she told me.

I was nervous about what Jack would think. He's the person I worry the most about seeing me like this.

'Well, did you see the paper?' I asked him on the phone.

'Yeah,' he said. I could tell he was smiling. 'You look great, it really suits you.'

I felt so relieved.

I remember years ago meeting Gail Porter just

after she lost her hair to alopecia and stress. She went out there with no wig or headscarf and I told her how brave she'd been.

No one knocked her for it and I am sure it will be the same for me.

At the end of the day I don't want my kids to be embarrassed by my baldness. I don't want them to think that if you're bald you have to hide away. They need to know it's okay. There are so many people out there with cancer and alopecia who can't wear wigs because they have allergic reactions to them, so my kids have to learn that having no hair is a part of life for some people.

Maybe I'll get some stick for whacking my bald head at people in their Sunday newspaper, but who cares? I don't want to be worried that people are staring at me as I'm walking round Tesco and doing the school run. I'd rather confront it head on (ha, ha!). Anyway, I've had to learn to laugh at myself over these past few years, before anyone else gets a look in. It takes away the pain of being laughed at if you do it yourself first.

*   *   *

I went curtain shopping afterwards. Nothing like a bit of retail therapy to sort you out.

20th January 2009

Carried on with my DIY today. I painted my bathroom pink and put a black chandelier in there to top it off. Jack will probably hate it but I love it. Freddy, who loves Cinderella, called it his

149

Cinderella bathroom! He is so funny.

I painted it pink while wearing a pink T-shirt. The Living crew said they merged together and it looked on screen like I was just a bald head floating around! It cracked me up.

I'm feeling a bit brighter today and thought of the first monthly activity I'd love to do with my girls. When we're all free I want to book the Pineapple Dance Studio and learn a dance routine to that song 'Baby Got Back' by Sir Mix-a-lot. Then we can go to Covent Garden, sling a hat on the ground and perform it! With a bit of luck we'll be good enough to earn a bit of money for a drink afterwards.

22nd January 2009

Mum was approached by *The People* to do an interview. She asked me first and I said okay. I hate people selling stories on me right, left and centre but it's different when it's Mum. I thought it might be good for her to talk about how she's feeling about my cancer. Maybe it will help.

Danny was going with her. Before they left, I said to him: 'Don't let her talk about this, don't let her talk about that. I don't want my medical records and chat about my poo with doctors and stuff going in that newspaper!'

He knows what my mum's like. No subject is off limits. She once made up a story that she used to wash my face in wee and it haunted me for ages.

Anyway, Mum says it's gonna be emotional so I'm glad I won't be there to watch! Hope it helps her feel better letting it out. I know watching all this is so tough on her. I want her to get her side of things across but I couldn't help feeling a bit nervous as I watched her going off in the car . . .

24th January 2009

Had lunch in Prezzo's in Epping with the girls and we had a right giggle. They all say I look really young with my new bald head. I was supposed to go out to see *Bride Wars* with Jen's sister Angela afterwards, but I was too tired. I really wanted to see it though. I love wedding films.

25th January 2009

Got teary reading Mum's interview with *The People*. I love her so much and know how much she loves me. She has been brilliant over the last few months—such a support to me.

I have completely forgiven her now for what she did when I was younger. And I want to make peace with my dad. He's dead now, so why should I still hate him for the things he did when I was young? I've let go of all that because of my illness. I feel all new inside.

Mum really does the best she can but I still don't think she knows how sick I am. She doesn't understand statistics or what a 40 per cent survival rate means. (*This is the latest I'm being told. Why is it going down rather than up?*)

I popped over to Mary's house and saw Louis. We watched some funny wedding dances on YouTube. There was a hilarious one where this

151

couple suddenly started doing a funky dance without any warning.

'Ha ha ha!' I screamed. 'Can you imagine Jack doing that? I want to do this at my wedding one day.'

Later on Kel and I went round to Jen's flat to watch a DVD. They asked me to bring some popcorn so I bought this massive giant tub with four different types. Jen put on *Seven Pounds* with Will Smith. We didn't realise it was about a little girl who dies and I sobbed all the way through.

Jen kept asking: 'Do you want a tissue?' And I kept saying no. But it upset me quite a lot.

26th January 2009

Awful news today. Bob Coleman died of a heart attack. I can't stop crying. How could this happen? He was right as rain a couple of weeks ago. I'll miss him so much. He was like a surrogate dad, friend, businessman, so much to me. He'd been with Carole since she was fourteen so I don't know how she'll cope.

Poor Bob. He was only sixty-two. I'm in bits. How can this happen?

He really cared for me and we met up as often as we could. I can't believe it. I *didn't* believe it at first because Mum heard the news by text and she often gets texts wrong, but I checked up and it's definitely true. Poor old Bob. Poor Carole.

*   *   *

Tonight I'm staying in a hotel near Wayland Prison

as we're going to pick up Jack tomorrow morning and I want to be the first to throw my arms around him.

I made the boys chicken nuggets and chips for dinner, one of their favourites. They are well excited about Jack coming out. I told them the lions and tigers don't need him in the jungle any more.

Feeling a bit nervous about seeing Jack. I've been through so much since we last spent time together. I know he loves me but I'm scared about what's going to happen. He's gone through one life-changing experience in there and I've been through another out here. Since he's been inside I've had operations, lost my hair, and chucked up almost every single night so I've lost tons of weight. I'm not the same girl I was when he went in.

People think he's a bad lad, but here is a boy who has never so much as touched a cigarette even when he was in prison, surrounded by drugs, cigarettes and god knows what else.

His mum told me she's been warned he might get depressed because when prisoners are released it's a bit of an anticlimax.

I just thought: 'Well, he'd better not!'

He's free now but I'm not—I've still got cancer. If he gives me grief over anything I won't have it. Not this time. I have changed. I've decided that if he puts a foot wrong then he's out. I've been through the worst time of my life and know I can do it on my own if I have to. I do love him but any more messing and that will be it.

We all set off in our big cars—me, Mary, and Kate with her film crew. It looked like a convoy of important people, like prime ministers or something! I told Kate she had to join all the paps as it's not fair putting Jack on camera as soon as he walks out the prison gates. She wouldn't make a very good pap, though, as she got lost and had to ring me up to find out where I was!

Mary and I had a lovely evening, chatting over dinner in the hotel. I had a chicken salad but it wasn't very nice. Nothing tastes good any more—it all tastes of metal.

I went to bed at 10pm and left Mary chatting to Kate. I sent Mary a long text after I got into bed: 'Tomorrow is a great day, the start of a new beginning. I can't wait, I bet you can't either. Have a good sleep and look forward to the morning. Lots of love to you xxx oh the beds are so comfortable xxx.'

Chapter Fourteen

My Jack Comes Home

27th January 2009

Had a terrible night last night—up, down, up, down, chucking up my guts. I swear the people in the hotel room next door must have thought I had a man in here with all the groaning going on.

The excitement of seeing Jack again took over as I got ready early. I put on a lovely white outfit and boots I knew he'd like. I wonder what he'll think of my bald head in the flesh? Hope he likes it. Well, tough if he doesn't!

The Living crew interviewed me in the hotel and I told them that one of the side effects of the radiotherapy is that it makes your la-la close up. The doctors wanted to give me a glass tube to help re-open that place, but sticking things up myself is not my thing. I told them that I'd rather have Jack do it. Can't believe I said that on camera. Me and my big gob!

When he walked out, his mum ran over and hugged him first, then it was my turn. He gave me a right smacker on the lips.

'I love you,' he whispered.

For once my tummy felt all like butterflies, instead of sick. *Jack is coming home! He is home!*

We went straight to Toys R Us and Jack bought a monkey for Freddy and a crocodile for Bobby, the animals he told the boys he'd been looking after in Africa. Then we picked them up from school together. They were over the moon to see him.

Jack took them straight out to play football in the garden. It felt so good to be all together again. He's still got to wear his tag and be at his mum's house every night for curfew at 7pm, as though he is an animal or something.

But at least I get my gorgeous boy back during the daytime.

I missed my chemo at the hospital today, but it was worth it to see Jack. *I love him so much. I'm so happy he's back.*

28th January 2009

Jack went to a beauty salon this morning to get a tan because he looked so white coming out of prison. I miss my brown boy! He says he looks like a ghost.

I went with him to the salon but afterwards he went off with some of his friends to get something to eat. I didn't mind him hanging out with them for a bit. He needs to adjust back into the real world.

He's relieved the strain of prison is over for me and I don't have to worry about phone calls or visiting any more.

'We can just be together now,' he says.

I don't feel too good today. The pains have started again and I feel a bit sick.

I spent some lovely time with the boys, watching them kicking a ball around with Jack, and then went to Mary's house to stay overnight. But as soon as I got there I threw up. The pain is so bad.

'It's killing me, Jack, this is bollocks,' I said.

I kept getting up and down all night long. I never let him see me in the bathroom, though. A girl has to keep her dignity somehow.

I am dreading going to the Marsden tomorrow as I don't want any more treatment. I've still got all the side effects from last time: sickness, ulcers and blisters in my mouth, and the terrible tiredness. Can I really face letting them put more of that poison in?

But I have to. I have no choice. *God, I hope this is all worth it.*

29th January 2009

Jack came with me to the Marsden for my chemo. In the taxi on the way there we had to stop so I could be sick.

When we got there they ran some tests and decided I was too ill to have chemo today. To be honest I was glad. I couldn't face it.

But I'm bloody miserable because they want to admit me for a while for tests. What's more, they've referred me to the Surrey Marsden for a scan because there weren't any beds at the London one. I don't want to go there as it's so far away from everyone.

Then I heard that there's a picture in the paper of Jack and his friends with their bums hanging out. He says they just flashed their white bums in an alleyway after the tanning session and a photographer caught them. He thought it was funny. Why does he always have to do it? His girlfriend is really ill and he goes around making an arse of himself?

I don't want him to sit with me in hospital all the time. He needs to go out with his mates and have fun too. Anyway, he has to get back for his curfew at 7pm.

I felt miles away from anywhere when I got out to Surrey. I know people at the London Marsden and they know me. It's like my security blanket. The pain can't get me when I'm in there.

Apparently some legal people have been saying in the papers I could sue the NHS because they didn't spot the warning signs of cervical cancer. In the past I've had smear tests which showed abnormal cells. Even though I kept collapsing and bleeding heavily no one put two and two together. So for years this sick disease was growing inside of me and nothing was done.

But I don't care what people tell me, I won't be suing anyone. The NHS is for everyone and if I took them to court for money, others would go without. Of course, it would be good if somewhere along the line lessons can be learned. I'd hate to think of any other mum going through this nightmare. But for now I just have to focus on getting better and I don't want to think about anything else.

30th January 2009

I don't like being here. I miss the boys but I don't want them to visit because I don't want them to see me this ill.

Mum was by my side non-stop over the last couple of days, keeping me sane, stroking my bald head, but she left yesterday to go and see Carole (Bob's wife) in Bristol, taking the boys with her. Kate drove them down.

Jack managed to pop in and see me this afternoon and I got a much-needed hug. I didn't want to let his hand go. I've had hardly any time alone with him since he got out because of the stupid curfew but I don't really want to see anyone else. I want to be on my own.

*   *   *

Then the doctors came round after he left and told me the results of the latest scan. I could sense from

158

their faces it wasn't good.

'Your cancer has spread to your bowel, liver and lymph nodes in your groin,' they said.

I started shaking. 'No!' I yelled.

After all this! All the bloody chemo and hospital visits. This couldn't be right. When is someone going to give me a fucking break?

'How long have I got?' I asked.

The doctors said it hasn't come to that. Just because one type of chemo hasn't worked doesn't mean another won't. There are still lots of options. They weren't prepared to give up hope and, of course, neither am I. There is no way on earth I am leaving Bobby and Freddy. This is just another setback.

'Right, what next then?' I asked.

My team explained the next step.

I am going to have a two-month course of a chemo drug called Hycamtin, also known as topotecan. It's from a Chinese tree. I never thought my life could depend on a tree!

'Okay, let's do it!' I said. 'Let's get started.'

*   *   *

After they all left I started crying and rang my mum in Bristol. I had to call a few times before she picked up.

'Mum, why don't you pick up your phone?' I said.

'Hello, Jade,' she said. 'I am just in the garden, playing with the boys.'

'Mum,' I said. 'It's all spreaded [sic]. It's all over me. My bowels, liver, groin . . .'

I heard a bang and a pause before Kate picked

159

up the phone.

'Jade? Your mum just fainted . . . we'll call you back,' she said.

'Look after her, Kate, please. She'll need it. My cancer has spread. They can't stop it.'

In the background I could hear Freddy trying to wake Mum up. 'Wake up, Nanna,' he was shouting. He thought it was that game they always played when she pretended to be dead.

'Look after her, Kate,' I repeated.

'We're going to drive straight home now,' she said.

I hope my mum doesn't cry too much and upset the boys. I need her to be strong.

31st January 2009

Decided to discharge myself. I have my painkiller pump and know how to work it, so fuck it.

Mary and Jack drove me back to theirs. The boys are with my mum.

I felt freezing, as I was only wearing a thin top. Jack had bought me a fleece dressing gown and new, warm pyjamas so I put them on. We sat in his bedroom and talked and cuddled.

He is so upset. He really believed it was only a short time before I got better. So did I.

'I thought this couldn't get any worse,' he kept saying, 'After all that chemo and stuff.'

I want to stop him from hurting and I can't. I hate seeing the sadness on his face.

He is still being positive, though, everyone is. So am I. There is no option in this for me. I have to get better as soon as possible. The doctors are going to help me. I will try any drug going to get there. I don't care what it's made from—trees, flowers, slugs, snails—you name it, I'll try it!

*   *   *

Jack and I went off to see the boys and have a play with them. Just seeing them makes it all go away and gives me certainty that more can be done.

I gave them their bath and put them to bed, then went back to Jack's house to stay.

The pain was so bad today I am struggling.

Mary cooked me dinner—jacket potato, salad and chicken. I've still got nasty pains but managed to eat it. Then I took myself off to bed around 8.30pm.

I woke up and went downstairs and Mary had made a lovely-looking apple crumble, so I ate a bit and felt horrible pains again.

I started being sick all night and didn't stop. God knows what was in my tummy. I kept thinking I had nothing left but still I was throwing up. I am wondering how this is all going to end. *When will it stop? What on earth is happening to me?*

Chapter Fifteen

From Bad to Worse

1st February 2009

The pain was so so bad. I was chucking up early this morning and Mary woke up.

'I am sorry to have woken you,' I said.

'Don't be silly,' she told me, then she said: 'Jade, I think we should go back to the hospital.'

Everyone wants to help and no one can do anything. Nothing seems to stop this terrible pain. I'd do anything for it to stop.

'I'll get an ambulance,' I said, but Jack and his mum insisted they would drive me. I hate putting people out like this.

Jack was due to take Bobby out for the day today. I knew he'd be disappointed to miss it.

'Babe,' I said. 'Look after Bobby for me. He'll be gutted if he misses you.'

Jack wanted to come with me, but I insisted. 'Do it for Bobby.' I said. 'Keep things normal.'

When we got outside I realised it had been snowing in the night and everything was white and frosty. They got me in the car and Mary and I drove to the Royal Marsden. I know the way so well now.

I was trembling by the time we got there because of the agony.

'This is the first time I am properly scared,' I sobbed to Mary. 'None of this is fair.'

'No, it isn't,' she replied.

The nurses tried to put tubes down my nose and it was horrible. I wanted to scream. It felt as though I was suffocating. That didn't work so they gave up and gave me painkillers. They must have been strong ones because before long I felt woozy and that horrible pain had gone.

*   *   *

One of the nurses brought a sack of letters to my

bedside that people had sent to me care of the hospital. Whenever I have a low moment (and there are lots of those right now), kind letters from the public keep me going. I've had some amazing ones.

It's heartbreaking that so many people have suffered with this evil disease. They all have their own ways of coping and getting on with it. They write to me with all kinds of ideas on how to get better. They send bottles of blessed water, bibles, flowers. Every single letter is opened and read, I try and make sure of that. I'd love to answer them all because they're so nice but I have no energy at all. I feel like a flat battery.

I started dozing off before long and told Mary she could go. She's been amazing to me. There aren't many people I can stand to spend time with just now but she is definitely one of them.

2nd February 2009

When the drugs wear off, the terrible pain comes back again.

I really don't want to see anyone. Have switched my phone off. Mum is doing her best to help but there is nothing anyone can do.

Charlene turned up today.

'What you doing here?' I shouted. 'I said no visitors.'

'I came to see you,' she said.

'Fine, now you've seen me you can go,' I said.

And she did.

I don't want to feel like I have to entertain people, or talk, or make jokes. I just want to be alone.

Someone told me there is snow everywhere, the first snow in years. I thought of the boys and how excited they must be.

They are with Jeff just now and I'm sure he'll take them out in it.

4th February 2009

Charlene came to visit again. She's so good, popping in and out, getting stuff for me when I need it and not minding if I snap at her. She is such a good friend.

I like talking about normal things when my friends are here. I want to know what they're doing, how their work is, what their boyfriends are up to. I don't want to sit here and talk cancer all day long.

Charlene has seen me through so much. She was there with me when I was pregnant with Freddy and went into false labour, and when I had my boobs done. And now this.

Never in a million years did either of us ever imagine this.

It came out in the papers today about my condition having spread to bowel, liver and groin. People know now. For once I don't ask what the articles are saying. It doesn't matter to me one way or the other.

5th February 2009

Someone sent me a copy of the *American Bible* and I decided to flick through it. Straight away I came to these words in Jeremiah 33: 'Call to me and I will answer you. I will tell you wonderful memories, things you know nothing about.'

It seemed like a message that was put there just for me to find. It was kind of spooky.

I've started to read passages out to people but I don't always understand what they mean and need help with some of the words. It's comforting stuff though.

My mum and dad were never religious, so I don't know where I got this from. Mum had a bible in the house but I don't think she read it. Before and after every mealtime, she told me to pray and thank God for the meals we had (she does this with Bobby and Freddy now). Right from the beginning I made up my own prayers—about whatever I wanted at the time mostly.

I do really believe in God and always have. Reading more of the Bible and trying to understand what it means is taking quite a lot of my time.

*　　　*　　　*

Jack comes to visit and stays with me for as long as he can before he has to go back for his curfew. We have a giggle. There's a trainee doctor who comes in and really makes us laugh because she just agrees with everything you say! Whatever anyone says she nods her head and says: 'Yes, yes.'

It cracks us up.

There's another doctor whose breath is so bad I can't help but turn my head away when he starts chatting.

Jack tries not to laugh and that sets me off.

Honestly, I am not just being mean. It really is that whiffy.

6th February 2009

I was in absolute agony this morning. I can't go to the toilet properly. It's disgusting to think what is stuck up there.

All I can think of is the pain. I just hold my stomach, crying, doubled up in pain.

The doctors have decided I need another operation straight away to get rid of the blockage. I can't stand it any more. They told me they could give me a colostomy bag that my poo would go into but I begged them not to. That's the last thing I need. I'd never feel like a woman again.

*   *   *

I woke up after the operation feeling like crap, but at least the pain has gone.

The doctors told me they found a golf ball-sized tumour blocking my bowel but they can't remove it all. They've done a by-pass to stop the blockage and that's all they can do.

I can actually feel the tumours through my skin, I think. I told my friends I have ten tumours but afterwards found out that was wrong.

Mum turned up later asking where Jack was. She looked well annoyed when I said he wasn't

166

here. She'd been waiting for him to ring her and let her know when I went down to theatre so that she could come in and I wouldn't be on my own when I woke up after the operation. I think he forgot, or there was a misunderstanding or something. Anyway, she is hopping mad at him.

7th February 2009

Recovering from the bowel op, I feel like I've been run over by a truck.

Jack turned up with his dad this afternoon after doing some filming with Kate in the morning. I was pleased to see him but Mum wasn't. There was real tension in the air between them.

To change the subject, I showed Andy my thumb pulse wire. It beeps when my heart beats but keeps slipping off. Annoying thing.

'Let's see your pulse then,' I said, giving it to him.

He put it on and his heartbeat is really slow because he does so much exercise. Suddenly all the alarms went off on the monitor and the nurses came rushing through thinking I was having a heart attack.

'It wasn't me, it was him,' I said, laughing. 'It's because he's fit and does things like football, running and picking mushrooms.'

After they left, Mum was still very angry with Jack. She felt he'd let me down. Thing is, he had to get back last night for his curfew. I know he would have stayed if he could.

I could hear the upset in her voice. 'Just leave it, Mum,' I said. 'Leave it, for god's sake.'

I hate it when Mum and Jack fall out. I was fuming. I just didn't want any hassle. There were more important things to worry about.

8th February 2009

A priest came to visit me and gave me a crucifix that will never leave my side, and I got some holy water.

I also saw a healer. I wasn't sure anything he could do would work but I couldn't see any harm in trying.

He placed his hands all over me, and it was really soothing. I'd not been able to go to the loo since my operation, but after the healer left I managed a number two. So that was a result for healing! It was a big relief and means I can carry on with the treatment now.

A lot of people say there's no point in looking into stuff like healing but I always like trying different things and it's made me want to try more. It just felt really nice to be relaxed for once.

My agent, Mark, had a call from Tara Palmer-Tomkinson offering to pay for me to visit Prince Charles's therapist! I am not sure exactly what kind of therapy he would give me but I am up for any kind of holistic treatment.

I also plan to start yoga and meditation.

*   *   *

It looks as though my feud with Katie Price is over once and for all. After realising how ill I am, she apologised for giving me a hard time for talking about my cancer to magazines. She says I am welcome around hers for tea and a chat. I'm not sure how that can happen now she lives in the States but I'd like to keep in touch. I'm glad we're not rowing but does she have to keep talking about it all?

*   *   *

Andy came and sat with me for a bit this afternoon. I like chatting to him. We decided that we must actually be living in hell, and because I've been good I've only got twenty-seven years. Andy must have been bad because he has had fifty years so far.

It was a funny conversation that made me think a lot afterwards.

*   *   *

Mum took the boys to London for the day. She showed me pictures afterwards. They went to Buckingham Palace to see the changing of the guards.

Bobby said 'Give me five!' to a policeman and he looked down and said: 'Oh, you're one of Jade's boys!'

He let them have a seat on his horse and sorted them out to get the best view for the changing of the guards ceremony.

Mum brought me a lovely shot of them wearing police helmets in their raincoats.

I am glad they are away from all of this, having fun.

9th February 2009

It was Bob's funeral today in Bristol. I wanted to go but obviously I can't. I am too ill. Poor Bob. Neither of us had any idea just a few weeks ago we'd be in these positions.

Sometimes I am glad we don't have crystal balls. It would be much worse to know what was coming.

10th February 2009

Another pile of post arrived today. I can't believe how it's all mounting up. I open as much of it as I can. I've already ordered my friends to reply to every single letter.

People are so thoughtful. One woman wrote to say how I'd helped her be proud of her own bald head by showing mine off. There's nothing to be ashamed of, is there?

It's not just letters either. I've had some lovely gifts. Someone made me a bracelet with B and F written on it.

I cried when I opened another handwritten letter and parcel from a little nine-year-old girl. She told me how she'd been abused by a family member, but there was something special that helped her and she thought that it might help me. I opened a Tupperware box, covered with tissue, and in it was a small stone.

'Rub this stone when you are feeling sad,' she wrote. 'It has helped me through my own hard times.'

I showed the girls that one when they came to

visit and we were all really touched.

*   *   *

I like some of the nurses. There is a camp one called Alex who I adore.

But my sense of smell has gone mad—I found out today it's one of the side effects of the treatment. Now I can smell anyone a mile off.

As one nurse was leaning over me getting some medicine, I wrinkled my nose to Kate.

'God, someone give her some chewing gum,' I said.

Mum came in and I nearly retched.

'Urgh, Mum, take that perfume off—it stinks.'

'But it's your perfume,' she said.

'I don't care,' I said. 'It's just too strong for me now.'

Is there a single bit of my body that isn't affected by all this? I've lost weight, my hair's gone, my mouth's got ulcers, even my feet are getting covered in horrid hard skin. I can't think of anything that's the same as it used to be before this started.

My voice. That's it! I've still got my big loud voice!

Chapter Sixteen

Time Is Running Out

11th February 2009

Dr Ind came to see me on his own this morning. I remembered what he'd said about one-to-one straight talking and decided I wanted some answers.

He said hello first and asked me how I was.

'What do you really think about things?' I asked.

He said quietly: 'I think you should be making arrangements for your children.'

I knew exactly what that meant and it made me feel sick to my stomach.

My boys would no longer have their mother because I won't be here . . . Oh my god. Oh my god.

Kate opened the door to come into the room and I screamed at her to get out and not to talk to Dr Ind.

'How long do I have?' I sobbed.

And he said: 'We don't know how long.'

'A year?' I asked

He shook his head and looked vague.

'Six months?'

He said he couldn't tell.

I am going to die from this but don't know how long I have left to live. Oh my god. How can this happen?

My head was spinning. So much to do. How would I tell Bobby and Freddy? How am I going to deal with this?

Mum came into the room and the look on her face said it all. She knew and we held each other.

'No! No! I'm devastated,' she kept crying. 'My baby . . .'

It broke my heart. I can't protect her from this. I can't help anyone with this pain.

How can this be happening? Is there really nothing anyone can do? I just can't believe it.

Kate came in, her face streaming with tears. She knew what had been said.

'I am so sorry, Jade,' she cried.

I tried to comfort Mum but I was crying so much I could barely see. Kate tried to as well. It felt like some kind of emotional bomb had gone off in our room. We were all clinging to the wreckage.

Nothing would ever be the same. I'd said all along I'd beat this, I had to for my babies, and yet the doctors have told me that cancer will end my life.

Mary arrived. When she came in I wiped my tears and said: 'I've had some bad news, but let's talk about something nice first.'

Of course, she looked white with shock. 'Just tell me, Jade,' she said. 'What's happened?'

'They've told me I'm going to die,' I said. 'It's spread. No one knows how long I've got. Maybe six months?'

She started crying too. I hate causing so much grief to so many people.

She rang Jack. 'You'd better come now,' she said.

When Jack arrived looking white as a sheet, so scared, I took his hand. 'Babe, I am not going to make this,' I said. His lips wobbled. 'It's not working. I think I have six months left now.'

He started crying and I tried to cuddle him. It was as if I could see his heart just shatter in front of me. I knew in that moment just how much he loved me.

'We'll do something,' he said, quickly. 'Some other doctors might be able to help you. Other treatments, something. Anything.'

I shook my head. 'Jack, they've done all they can. They tried.'

*   *   *

After Jack had to leave, I grabbed my phone and started ringing people. One by one I rang my friends.

I rang Jen's mobile and she was in a noisy bar.

'Sorry, Jade,' she yelled. 'I can't hear you!'

'It's bad news,' I said. I never say that, so that got her listening.

The sound of music died down as she went somewhere quieter.

'You what?' she asked.

'I have only got six left, Jen,' I replied. 'It's got me. I'm going to die.'

She was sobbing down the phone. I waited for her to calm down and listen.

'Don't cry,' I said. 'Please don't, for me.'

Jen, Kel and Caroline hurried in to visit me, looking really upset. They were in a terrible state and just trying to hold it together. At one point Jen left the room and I knew it was because she didn't want me to see her falling apart. Carefully I unhooked myself from one machine after another. I shuffled into the wheelchair I'd been using since the bowel op and pushed myself across the corridor to look for her.

I found Jen in a side room, tears dripping off her nose.

'Don't be sad,' I soothed. 'I'll be okay. I'm really going to miss you.'

We had a cuddle and she started crying worse than ever.

*   *   *

Jeff rang later to say Bobby was in his school play today as a DJ and that he'd videoed it for me. This is one of the first ones I have missed.

How do I tell them? How does a mummy tell her children such a thing?

I can't bear it.

*   *   *

Late at night I was transferred to the fifth floor, to the Horder ward where all the seriously ill people go. I joked around with the porters: 'If it's the fifth floor you know you're going to die. The floor of death, the floor of doom. Press the button to die.'

They laughed.

I do like some of the staff in here. There is a priest I really like. I call him Father Ted.

Everyone is in shock. So am I, to be honest. I just want to focus on getting home now.

12th February 2009

Jack did a shoot for *OK!* magazine today. I told him to do it. I wanted him to have a bit of fun and put his side of things across. He doesn't like the limelight like me, though.

'Jade, do I really have to?' he kept asking. He wasn't sure if it was the right time to be doing something like this.

'Look, it's more important than ever,' I said. 'Go! You have to make the most of it. Make as much money as you can out of the mags.'

But he says all the money will go to the boys. Despite what people think, he hates living off my fame.

I laughed when he texted me to say he hated the clothes and shoes they'd given him to wear. Mark was with him and he took photos on his phone and sent them to me, so I sent back some advice about what to wear with what.

Mark and Jack thought it was funny that even from a hospital bed 15 miles away I could still boss everyone around.

My solicitor came to talk about my will. I want to set up a trust fund for the boys. He told me I need a board of trustees to look after it and straight away I thought I'd like Kate, Simon and Danny. I'll have to ask them. We didn't finish but it's a start. Things have to start happening now, preparations have to be made. I want everything to be in place.

*   *   *

Later on Kate said she'd stay the night and I was

glad. I wanted someone to be close. As she lay on her camp bed, mouth hanging open, she made me snigger.

'Are you falling asleep like that? You look really weird,' I said, winding her up.

'Sssh,' she said. 'I'm knackered.'

'So what?' I said, knowing she'd been running round after me all day. 'I have a few more things for you to sort out in this room before you drop off.'

She shook her head.

'Get up,' I teased.

'If you don't shut up I'll pull your drip out,' she snapped.

I giggled. So glad she was there. We're not filming any more, obviously, but she'll be around for whatever I need her to do. She's an amazing friend.

I lay in the quiet, thinking. I couldn't drop off. I kept seeing dark shadows climbing round the walls, looking like people. It frightened me so I buzzed for the nurse.

'Is this what happens when you die?' I asked. 'Do shadowy people in the corner come and take you away?'

'No,' said the nurse, gently. 'You just know, you have feelings. People won't come and take you.'

I looked up at her. 'Do you pray, nurse?' I asked. 'Will you pray for me tonight?'

'Of course I will,' she said, and kissed me on the head.

I wakened Kate in the middle of the night when the tears came again. 'This is torture, Kate. This is so cruel, just waiting to die. I want the nurses to give me something. I want you to take me to

America. They let people die in America.'

'Do you mean Switzerland?' Kate asked.

'Yeah, Switzerland,' I said. 'Yes, that's what I mean.'

She said we could talk about it in the morning but right then I should try and get some sleep. She was right. She always knows best.

13th February 2009

This morning I did an interview with the *News of the World* in which I told them I was dying. Mark was there, and Kevin came along too. I caught hold of both of their hands and said: 'Mark, promise me one thing. Promise me you will make Kevin a gladiator!'

He'd be a wicked gladiator!

Mark said he would do his best.

*   *   *

I just don't want to write what happened next. I can't bear it. How much does one person have to take?

This afternoon some nurses and the matron were gathered next to my bed, sorting out medication, making sure I was comfortable.

I am so tired I trust them to do as much as they can. But I just wanted to know the truth now. I've got so much to prepare for my kids that I need to know what's going to happen to me next.

'I need to know what I need to know and now,' I began.

The matron looked confused. I looked at Kate.

'She means she wants to know how long she

178

has,' she said.

'How long have I got?' I asked. I was thinking six months at least because Dr Ind didn't contradict me when I suggested that the other day.

'Do you really want to know?' the matron asked kindly. 'Are you sure?'

'Yes,' I said. 'Yes, tell me, I do.'

'One to two months,' she replied, softly.

I tried to take a breath but the air wouldn't go in.

A horrible animal sound came from nowhere— and it was coming from my mouth.

'Noooooooooo!' I screamed, tears just pouring out of me. 'Noooooooooooooooo.' I just wanted to howl and cry and scream. I held my head in my hands to try and take it in. 'What about my babies? What about them?' I screamed. 'No!'

Kate climbed onto the bed to lie next to me as I sobbed.

'Can't anyone do anything?' I screamed. I looked at their poor faces. 'Can't anyone help me? Can't you?'

A couple of weeks ago when they first told me the cancer had spread they said it didn't have to be the end. There were lots of other medicines out there and things to do.

I really believed them. Believed I'd be okay. I had to be for my boys.

Then after the bowel op, a little part of me worried I wouldn't get better. I felt so bloody ill. Then I was told it was terminal but I didn't know how long. Somehow I could handle all that, but not this. *Not this. Not one or two months.*

* * *

I started to try and sort myself out. I had to tell people. I had so much to do. *Oh my god. Every second is so precious now.*

I grabbed Kate and started talking at top speed (and that's fast!). 'Sort out the insurance, the houses, pay the bills, talk to Danny and Simon about being trustees for the boys, look after my mum—I know she'll drive you bonkers but look after her—and my nan and granddad.'

I knew I had to let the family know.

'I want my mum,' I cried. 'I want my mum.'

Someone started dialling Mum's number.

They all came. I don't know how or when, but suddenly lots of people were by my side. My mum was shaking with tears, trying to cuddle me, sobbing. Mary was crying as well.

'Can't someone just give me something if I have to die?' I cried. 'Can't I have a pill to kill me? Can't I be put out of my misery?'

Mum held me as I sobbed and sobbed.

The nurses said they couldn't help, that it had to happen bit by bit.

I was dying now. I am twenty-seven and I am dying. Oh God.

*   *   *

I rang Jeff and told him I only had weeks left to live. 'We've got so much to do to sort out the kids.'

He was stunned.

It was like any ill feeling between us during the years was just swept away in a second. All our petty rows and arguments really had meant nothing. We had our kids, we both loved them and

180

wanted the best. I knew he'd try his absolute best to help.

'Can you bring the boys in?' I asked. 'I really need to see them. Please.'

He agreed that he would.

*   *   *

Jack showed up soon afterwards, his face so worried.

'All that chemo, all that pain for nothing,' he cried. 'I won't accept this. I am not having this, Jade. We'll go to America. They always have new treatments. Some miracle cure we don't know about. We'll save you. We have to.'

I started crying again. I knew it was too late. 'I can't fly in this state, can I, Jack?' I lifted up my arm with all the tubes attached. 'It's too fucking late.'

I think Jack was in denial about a lot of my illness because he'd missed so much of it when he was in prison. He still expected the chemo to work, for me to get better, for us to have a family.

'We just have to make the best of it,' I said.

He took a deep breath and said: 'Right then, we're getting married. You're a special woman, I love you and I want to call you my wife.'

I managed to smile, a big happy smile.

Oh God. I'd just been told the worst news ever and now I was smiling?

'Are you sure you don't mind being a widow?' I asked.

Jack looked confused. 'Well, I won't be one, will I?'

'You know what I mean—after?'

181

'It doesn't matter,' he said.

'Let's get married then,' I said.

*   *   *

I haven't seen the boys for ages. I miss them so much. When they finally burst into the room I couldn't stop hugging them and smelling their hair. My two little bombs of energy. I only wished I felt stronger today. I am so tired and weak.

I talked to them gently.

'Do you like living with your dad?' I asked.

Bobby looked at me. 'No, we want to live with you.'

I carried on, trying to breathe. 'But you like living with your dad too, don't you? You have so much fun.'

'Yeah, we do,' said Bobby.

And then I couldn't tell them. It was all too much for one day. How do you say 'Mummy's going to die'?

Jeff put on the DVD of Bobby in his school play and we watched it together. He looked so pleased to be on stage.

'You were fantastic in that, Bobby,' I grinned, reaching for him.

We had a cuddle. Then we read a story together and played for a bit.

Even just lying here takes it out of me.

*   *   *

Jen, Kel and Charlene arrived and set up a picnic in the day room next door with sandwiches from the canteen. Bobby and Freddy ate their lunch and started darting around, in and out of the room. Their little faces were glowing. I so badly wanted to sit up more.

As they ran around, laughing, I suddenly felt a terrible pain, but this time an emotional one. The room swam with tears so I called for the girls.

'Please get them out of here,' I whispered.

They quietly shut the day-room door as they realised I couldn't hold back.

'I can't do this any more,' I cried, sobs rising in my chest.

In that moment I knew I couldn't be a proper mum to Bobby and Freddy any more. They were too much. I was too ill to look after my own kids.

It was over. My role as a mummy to the boys was finished. I am never going to feel better.

'I can't look after my own children any more! Why was I given something I love so much for it to be taken away? Why is this happening to me? I'm a good person. I've looked after my mum when I was a kid, I've looked after my friends, my boyfriends, my two boys! Why has this happened? Why has God given me something I love so much and then taken it away?'

The girls stood in silence, listening. Tears were everywhere. I knew it was upsetting for them to hear me like this but I didn't care. Suddenly I felt absolutely furious and I had to let it out.

*   *   *

Danny and Si came over in the evening, both of them crying. Everyone was in shock, horrified.

'Don't go out to a restaurant tonight,' I murmured. 'Get a takeaway, a KFC or something.'

They brought a big bucketful back. The nurse popped in and said I shouldn't be eating that. It wasn't good for my bowels.

'Fuck it,' I said, and took a big bite.

I started barking orders big time. Kate frantically scribbled a list in her diary, because she hadn't had time to get a notebook.

'You, Dan, Si can be part of my boys' trustees. The boys need a car each when they're eighteen. All the school bills need paying.' I was gabbling away. Every second mattered now, every precious hour.

My mind was in a whirl.

I turned to my girlfriends.

'I want all of you—Jen, Kel, Caroline, Kate and Charlene—to be my bridesmaids and that means you have to organise the wedding for me. Are you okay with that?'

They all nodded.

I started calling other friends too. I rang and spoke to Jen's mum, Sue, who I'd known for seven years.

Sue started crying and then passed me to Jen's sister Angela.

When she began crying I told her: 'Don't cry, life is for laughing.'

*　　　*　　　*

I hate this so much. None of this is fair. I want some answers. I want to look back over my life and find out what I've done wrong because this is bloody torture.

I can't be a mum any more and it's killing me.

Later Jen and Kelly stood in my room and

184

cuddled each other. I raised an eyebrow. Those two are not cuddly kinds of people at all and never hug everyone like I do.

They are always letting me cuddle them or play with their hair but don't themselves. It was lovely to see such affection between them.

'See,' laughed Kel. 'You've got us cuddling now.'

'You make sure you both keep doing it,' I said.

When everyone else left, Charlene set up her camp bed and slept next to me. I feel exhausted.

Chapter Seventeen

Planning the Wedding

14th February 2009

For Valentine's Day Jack got me a card that said 'To my Wife' and some flowers.

I didn't get him anything. I just feel too ill to think about it.

We hardly get a minute alone. So many people in and out, nurses, doctors, friends.

We watched a DVD—*Anchorman*—and cuddled.

My granddad and nan came in. No one had wanted to tell them the awful news on the phone so I had to tell them myself. It was the hardest thing I'd ever done.

Granddad was trembling as he sat down. I think he knew it was bad.

My voice went all croaky and weird. 'Granddad, I'm so sorry to tell you but I'm going to die in a few weeks,' I said.

His face just crumpled. Big sobs rose from his chest. I'm his only grandchild and will face death before him.

'This shouldn't be happening,' he said. 'I wish I could take your place.'

We held each other then he had to leave the room for a bit.

My nan is in the early stages of dementia and didn't seem to take it in.

Watching my loved ones hurt so deeply makes my own pain and fear even worse.

While all Mum's drug and police stuff was going on I always protected my grandparents from the truth. I didn't want to shatter their world so I'd go round there after school with a big smile on my face and pretend everything was fine. They adored me and I adored them. Now I've had to break their hearts.

This time I just couldn't shield them from the truth.

*   *   *

I told the boys—Simon, Danny and Kevin—to bring their wives for a little Valentine's Party this evening.

At 8pm I rang Kel to ask her where she was. 'You rang and told us not to come,' she said.

I had no memory of this. Must be the drugs talking. 'Well, get yourself down here,' I said.

Everyone arrived and brought loads of sweets—marshmallows and parma violets. I handed them out and then we put on *Forgetting Sarah Marshall*.

Kate tried to give me a foot massage but I was

embarrassed because the skin on my feet is all hard and cracked now. Horrible.

I felt so knackered, it was hard to be sociable. After the film finished I left the room and Kate followed me.

'I'm sorry, I can't do this,' I cried. 'I want people to go. I am just too tired to deal with them.'

'Don't worry, you don't have to,' said Kate.

She went back in and asked everyone to leave.

'Sorry I ruined your Valentine's Day,' I said as they left. 'Get yourselves off to the Embassy Club and have some fun. Have a drink on me.'

I rang Kel and told her not to come after all. I just want to sleep.

15th February 2009

I woke up this morning feeling full of energy for once. Charlene was with me.

'I want to tidy this place up,' I said.

We set to cleaning the whole room from top to bottom. I gathered up all the cards and papers. Charlene even cleaned the floor.

'I need fresh air in here,' I said, opening the window.

Jack arrived and seemed excited about something.

'Come on,' he said. 'You need to get your coat on.'

'Why?' I asked, as he got a wheelchair.

'We're going somewhere,' he replied mysteriously.

I grabbed Mary's coat and put on Louis' woolly hat. Someone said I looked like a refugee.

I felt a tingle of excitement. I hoped I knew what was coming.

The nurses were a bit worried about me going out. They said I shouldn't be long. I feel okay today, though. I want to do something normal.

The cold air felt good on my face and made me shiver. It was lovely to have some proper fresh air to breathe.

I used to feel sorry for people in wheelchairs but I don't mind Jack pushing me about. He says he likes taking care of me.

We went to Armani first to look at suits. Louis tried one on.

'How much is it going to cost?' I asked them. 'I want a discount because I am getting married and then I am going to die.'

The shop attendant was speechless.

Then Jack told his mum and Louis to leave. He carried on walking and walking and walking for ages, pushing me along in the chair.

'Where are you taking me?' I kept asking.

We arrived at a spot on the Thames, opposite Battersea Park.

He gave me a cheeky grin and then Danny and Simon showed up to warn us that the paps had been alerted. Loads of traffic was stopping and cameras were being pointed in our direction. Jack dropped on one knee.

'Jade, will you marry me?' he asked.

'Yes, of course,' I giggled, feeling a bit embarrassed.

We had a little kiss. 'Why do you want to marry me?' I asked.

'Because I'll be so proud to call you my wife,' he said.

188

He already had an engagement ring, from my mate Dave who does jewellery in Essex. It was a diamond and silver band.

It couldn't have been more romantic! It was just beautiful that he'd gone to so much trouble.

*   *   *

After that Jen, Kel, Caroline and Charlene turned up to take me shopping and Jack went off to do his boy stuff.

We went to Harrods and I tried on loads of wedding dresses. I loved every second of it even though it was tiring lifting up the heavy skirts. The one I picked was designed by Manual Mota and I'd thought I wouldn't like when I saw it on the rail but as soon as it slipped over my head I knew it was The One.

It cost £4K but when I went to pay, the assistants told me that Harrods were giving it to me. Isn't that kind? Their dress fitters will come and measure me in my hospital bed. It's tricky because I have a little bag with my pump and all my medicines in so have to make the dress fit around that. The girls call it my Gucci bag!

Ooh, I can't wait to be Mrs Tweed. Though I want 'Jade Goody' on my headstone because that's what people know me as.

Next I picked some gorgeous navy bridesmaids' shoes. They're Laboutins [sic!] with five-inch heels.

'What colour dress is going to go with them?' asked Jen.

'I dunno,' I laughed. 'It's not my problem, it's yours!'

189

Next we went to Selfridges and picked wedding rings for Jack and me from Tiffanys.

Simon had come along to take some pictures and he grabbed a bottle of champagne from the shelf and cracked it open.

'We're not stealing it really,' I said.

We'd been gone for hours and the hospital kept ringing my mobile.

'But I'm fine,' I kept saying, feeling like a teenager being told off for being out past my bedtime.

'Don't overdo it,' said the nurses. 'You need to come back. Your medication could run out.'

In the end they were threatening to call the police if I didn't come back. We only got peace and quiet when my mobile battery died.

We all piled into P.J.'s, the restaurant just outside the Marsden, for a late lunch.

Then the hospital rang someone else's phone and at that stage I thought I should probably go back so Jack wheeled me in.

'I'm sorry,' I said as the nurses rushed towards me. 'But I'm okay!'

Charlene stayed for a bit and we went through the guest list. I told her to ring all the mums I chat to in the playground at Bobby and Freddy's school. We agreed guests had to be rung and invited, but given no details of when or where. They'll be rung back later to confirm details and then back again for security details. It all has to be top secret because my agents are doing a magazine deal. Max is on TV the whole time talking about it and making sure the right message gets out.

I won't be inviting many celebs as I don't have many celebrity friends! I remember Katie Price invited me to her wedding. It was the most over-the-top invite I'd ever seen, all full of glitter. I didn't know her well, she wasn't a proper mate or anything, but we've always got on when our paths crossed. I couldn't go but I saw the magazine pictures and I thought she looked wicked on her big day. I just want people I am close to at my wedding, though.

Kel and Jen stayed the night on the camp bed next to me. I was so pleased to have them there.

Jen used to have a boyfriend whose mum was Irish and we'd always take the piss out of her accent. For some reason that came up and I started making them giggle with my impression. I think I'm great at accents, but Kel says I always sound Jamaican whatever one I try and do.

We just laughed a lot, which was good. Those two are so funny. When I was filming my show three years ago we all went skiing and the producers thought they were so funny, they called them Ant and Dec, and that nickname stuck.

They topped and tailed on the camp bed. Both are quite big girls.

'Is it uncomfy?' I kept asking.

Jen said she could smell something funny.

'I bet it's Kel's feet,' I cried. 'Your feet stink!'

During the night I kept getting waves of pain and had to press the buzzer for the nurse.

'Sorry, girls,' I kept saying.

Kel laughed. 'Will you stop being so selfish and pressing it, please?' she yawned.

Every time the nurse came in she'd accidentally knock into their bed.

Poor things were knackered.

We had such a giggle though. I love them so

191

much.

16th February 2009

I woke up in the morning to find a note from Jen and Kel: 'To Jen's ex-boyfriend's mum, Hope you got some sleep—we didn't, Love, Ant and Dec.'

It made me smile.

Mum says my half-brother Brett from Australia wants to contact me. I find that a bit suspicious. I hadn't heard from him when I was diagnosed, nor when I started going bald, but now I'm dying he wants to get in touch! I told Mark I don't want to see him.

Mum had him when she was young but he got put in foster care so I never really knew him. It's sad for her, but I've no interest in seeing him. I did meet him years ago and we didn't get on.

I have another brother called Miles but he doesn't know we're related. How sad is that? I had hoped to track him down one day but I doubt I'll have time now.

*   *   *

The boys went to get their suits fitted at Chris Kerr tailors in Soho. Danny uses him and has organised it. The poor bloke will have to work night and day to get them finished on time. It's so nice of him.

The bridesmaids went to Bluewater Shopping Centre to get their dresses. Kel and Jen told me that when they heard whose wedding it was for the shop assistants all stood around, gobs open, giving them champagne and strawberries and treating them like royalty. They texted me pictures of the dresses they chose. They're navy blue to match the shoes and I really like them.

Hope they're not having too much fun, though, as they've got loads to do. Get cracking, girls!

I could only look at a few things on my laptop because doing anything now makes me so knackered. I knew I could trust my girls to get stuck in and they did.

In the past, I'd always said my dream wedding would be going abroad for a quiet do, then coming back and having a massive party at the Savoy. I wanted a big tower of Ferrora Roche [sic] like in the telly advert. And my bridesmaids would be dressed in 1950s style and we'd all arrange a great dance.

That was all before I fell ill. Now I just want the biggest, best day we can plan in a week.

They've all got their own jobs to do. We've decided to have it in Down Hall Country House in Hatfield and Caroline is talking to them about the food. Today she sent up menus and Simon helped me choose what we would have.

There is so much to do. They're all taking time off work or just using their work phones to ring round.

I hope they manage it. I love my girls but have never seen them organise anything very well before! Even a simple get-together in a club can go pear-shaped with them in charge!

17th February 2009

Of all the things my name has been attached to, this one is unreal—smear tests! Kate told me that 20 per cent more women are getting them done now because of what's happened.

They are calling it the 'Jade Goody' effect.

Apparently some papers have done stories about women who found out they had cancer because of it. If any good is to come from this, that's great news.

The girls are so busy. I get phone calls all the time to check things. I know what I want and what I like.

Jack is helping too, but every time he tries to choose something he says: 'What's the point? You know what you want anyway.'

Harrods came to the hospital for a fitting. They put down a big sheet to stop the dress getting dirty.

My shoes were couriered over. They are so high. Hope I can walk in them as my feet are all dry and cracked now.

In the afternoon, Caroline came into the hospital room with an armful of Rob Van Helden flowers. He is being really sympathetic about all this because a friend of his died of cervical cancer, so it's close to his heart.

'These any good?' Caroline said, showing off beautiful blue and white ones of all different kinds.

'Yep,' I grinned.

The hospital say I can go home tomorrow. They have to work out if the drugs they have given me will manage my pain on the Big Day. If there are any problems I'll have time to change them before Saturday.

Chapter Eighteen

Home Sweet Home

18th February 2009

The hospital are so organised, they've been amazing. I have twelve different types of tablets, injections, and a drip permanently hooked up to my arm full of painkillers. My chemo has stopped for now. It won't be until next week that I'll know if it's going to start again.

The doctors came in and showed me my drug chart.

'Can you show Kate, please?' I asked, knowing she would understand it all better.

We packed up my room. I had loads of pictures stuck on the walls. Handprints from the boys. Photos of holidays with Jack. Pics of Mum and the boys pulling faces. And a collage I'd made for Jack's prison cell with all my fave pictures of us and some words written on it. He gave it back to me after he got out.

It was a bit scary leaving the hospital, where I have all the nurses and staff to help. I gave the paps a thumbs-up as the ambulance drove me off. I can't imagine what I look like, but don't care any more. I am still here—that's what counts.

Kate came with me in the ambulance but I have told her I don't want any more filming from now on. They can cover the wedding and that's it.

I don't need this any more.

I am home! Just smelling my familiar house smell as I was wheeled through my door made me happier.

Nurses will come round to keep an eye on me and make sure the pain isn't too bad. They will also help me to use the loo and sit in a chair for a shower. The doctors have told me to save all my energy and not walk around.

Mum and Jack had prepared the house. They shoved the dining room table to the side and put a hospital bed in there with all the equipment around it. Jack had put the Play-Station in there too so when the boys are here I can watch them playing.

Mary had bought me new white sheets and a lovely soft baby-pink fleecy blanket that I love.

I can see the rolling fields from the window, but the Shetland ponies aren't there any more. I don't know where they went. But it's still a lovely view.

Kate laid out all the drugs for me.

'Oh, bloody hell, Kate,' I said. 'Are you sure you know what you're doing?'

But she does. She's a smart girl.

The boys came for a visit in the afternoon. The hospital have given me a book about a badger who dies to try and explain to them what is happening.

I got out of my wheelchair and sat on the settee with them.

'Right, boys,' I said, taking a deep breath. 'It's time for us to look at this book the hospital gave me. Heaven is going to be calling me soon. I am going to be an angel and this book explains what will happen then. Would you like me to read it?'

Bobby frowned. 'You're alive so why do we have to listen to this now?' he said.

I stopped and looked at him then I closed the book.

'Do you know what, boys? You're right. I am alive.' I decided to read them a normal bedtime story instead. There should be time enough for the badger later.

*   *   *

The girls came to visit and we organised guest lists and I got into bride mode.

The nurse kept warning me not to overdo it but there was so much to do.

My girls all look exhausted with the hard work they've been putting in.

'You're an ugly bunch,' I laughed. 'You lot need a makeover.'

I told them to organise us some teeth-whitening and Botox.

'Botox?' said Jen. 'Do we really need that?'

I just cackled with laughter. I knew they'd love it really.

'Think of your pictures in the mag without the crows' feet,' I said, pointing them out on their faces. *OK!* are covering the wedding for £750,000. That's brilliant news for my boys.

Kate gave an interview to the *Mirror* today about the wedding and my illness. I wanted her to do it. She's insisting on putting the money into the boys' fund. She said: 'There are so many things to organise and so much of what Jade wants isn't practical when there is only a week—but if anyone can pull off this wedding, Jade can.'

Too right!

*   *   *

I wanted to stay up longer but the tiredness got the better of me and I had to go to sleep at 11pm.

The third instalment of my Living TV series hits the screens tomorrow. I quite like watching them myself, apart from the bits where I am crying. It makes me cry then!

I know some people think I shouldn't be showing all of this, but it helps me so I don't care. My illness is horrible and I'm glad if being open about it can do some good.

I've decided to let Living film my wedding. I need a wedding video anyway and they'll do a good job.

19th February 2009

Some of the girls popped in again. I hope they are not getting into trouble with their work.

'You lot are having a lot of time off,' I said. 'What is it—the credit crunch?'

At 9am a marquee was put up in my garden because we were going to have the reception there. Then Mark and Danny came in to see me while I was resting in bed and told me the marquee was coming down again. Talk about changing their minds! I was well annoyed.

'What the hell is going on?' I screamed. 'Just because I'm ill in bed doesn't mean you shouldn't let me know what's happening! It's my wedding after all!'

198

Mark explained that they'd had to explore three different reception venues because of Jack's tag. The first idea was to have it at Mary's house, but only about twenty people could fit into her garden. The second idea was to have it at mine, then it wouldn't be far for Jack to get home by 7pm, but then the guests would have to travel there after their meal at Down Hall. The third plan was that if Jack could get permission to get his tag off for one night, we could stay at the hall.

'Looks as though the probation people will let Jack off for the night,' said Mark. 'So we can take the marquee down.'

I stared at him. 'Alright,' I said. 'Just keep me informed.'

Then, later on in the day, we got the news that the probation officer had said there is no way Jack will get permission to miss his curfew. So now we don't know where to have the reception, which is a bit stressful to say the least.

The doctors came round to go through the drugs and pain relief and stuff but I didn't want to speak to them. I just avoided them. While they were there Kate arrived, looking really ill. They took one look at her clutching her tummy and sent her off to hospital. I hope it's not anything serious. Someone mentioned appendicitis, which would not be good news.

Then some man from a hospice came and suggested I should go and have a look.

I said no, today I am planning my wedding. I am not talking about dying.

Give me a flipping break from this.

*   *   *

Went to Loughton to get rings with the girls. I bought them each a silver platinum band and arranged for them to be engraved, saying: 'With you always, love Jade.'

I wanted to get Links of London friendship bracelets for Bobby and Freddy, but they didn't have the right colours so I ordered them.

Bishop Jonathan Blake came round to discuss our vows. Kev had suggested we use him.

'Do you want something traditional or sentimental?' he asked.

'What's best?' I asked. 'Because I'm dying.'

I couldn't read half the words he was showing us. In the end we agreed to repeat them after him so we don't get them wrong.

He asked us how we met. I told him it was in a nightclub and the first thing I thought about Jack was: 'God, you're fit!' My friend went over and gave him my number (which really embarrassed me), but he never rang. He'd read in the papers I'd got back with Jeff the following day, which was rubbish. So we only got together a few weeks later. When we met, Jack told me he was a twenty-two-year-old football agent. Turned out he was only eighteen and living at home with his mum and dad.

We've had some right ups and downs. The papers say he's only after me for my money, but I know what's what. Journalists have been writing articles wondering what I am going to leave him. Part of me thinks it's none of their business, but I am actually not leaving him anything. Everything is going to my boys. He doesn't want my money. I've offered to let him live in one of my houses if he pays the mortgage, but he doesn't want to. I have told Mark to organise an interview for him after I die so he could make some money from that—but then he doesn't like the spotlight so he might not even do it.

I still don't know what to do with my houses. In fact, I keep asking people: 'Do you want a house?' They always say no, they can't afford the mortgage repayments.

Anyway, the bishop asked what happened after Jack and I finally got together and I told him about how we were necking cocktails from a jug. So not that classy!

I love the words he has put together for our vows, though. They're beautiful. Exactly right!

*　　　*　　　*

I rang Kate in Harlow Hospital to see how she is. If she can't be a bridesmaid I will ask Carly, who I ran the beauty salon Ugly's with. But Kate seems to think she will manage.

'You need to paint your toenails navy blue if you have time,' I said. 'Just in case.'

I know she feels bad not being here as she was supposed to be helping me sort out my drugs. But the nurses will manage. I just want her to get better.

*　　　*　　　*

At 10.30pm the Botox doctor came to the house. He looked at my bridesmaids and said: 'They're stunning girls—they don't need any Botox.'

'Yes they do!' I said, grabbing Kel and showing him. 'Look at her forehead and eyes!'

'Jade!' said Kel, embarrassed.

They all agreed in the end and one by one had the needles. I held their hands because they were wincing.

'Come on, you can do it, just a few more seconds,' I said. What wimps! Needles don't bother me. I already look like a pincushion.

When it was her turn, Kel went white and nearly passed out. I was lying on the sofa but the doctor told me to give her my place.

'Your friend needs to lie down,' he said.

'Sorry, Jade,' Kel said. Honestly!

I can't eat much at the moment but I asked the girls to nip out and get me a chicken salad from Pizza Express. They tend to go down nicely.

I really wanted to stay up but the nurses kept warning me to go to bed and rest.

In the end I felt a bit weird and shivery and had to lie down. They call it a 'crash', seemingly. I don't remember much.

But it was a great night.

Charlene is going to stay over for a few nights now.

20th February 2009

The boys are back. So pleased to see them.

Mum came round bringing a toy lion that a well-wisher (she calls them wishing wells) gave her. She pressed the button and it sang 'Don't worry, Be happy . . .' in an annoying loud voice.

I looked at her and felt myself fill up with rage. 'Mum, turn that fucking thing off,' I snapped.

On and on and on this irritating music went.

'Turn it off. Now.'

Mum looked pale and tried to find the button but she couldn't! She picked it up and pushed its belly to try and switch off the damn noise and it carried on and on.

'Mum!' I shouted.

Then Freddy came running over and found the off button straight away.

'Sorry,' said Mum. 'Trust me.'

The bridesmaids went for another fitting. Their dresses had to be shipped in from Hong Kong and somehow the shop have managed to get it done in just three days even though they said at the beginning that it would take six weeks.

Jen walked in later with a big armful of tracksuits for us all—free gifts from Pineapple. She was well chuffed.

'God, you're getting good at this,' I said.

All my bridesmaids are getting offered freebies. Everyone wants to help when they hear it's for me, which is really nice of them.

*   *   *

I've invited Jeff to the wedding but he can't come because he is working as a presenter on the *X Factor* tour. I like the fact there are no issues between us now. It hasn't always been this way. We've had our rows about maintenance and time with the children. But he's been so good with Bobby and Freddy I have to forgive him. He even offered to buy me a wedding gift but I told him not to. All I want is donations for the boys' trust fund. Everything I have is going straight to my sons.

Jack won't be getting a penny out of the

wedding. Not because I'm being a bitch, but because that's what we both want. It's all for the boys.

*   *   *

Mary brought her friend Anne-Marie round to see me today. She's a Christian and I wanted to talk to her about getting the boys christened.

'Why don't you get christened too?' asked Anne-Marie.

'I thought only babies and kids could,' I replied.

'No!' she said. 'Adults too! If you want to, you can too.'

I smiled. In that case I will. I want to feel closer to God. I can do this one last thing for my boys.

*   *   *

I fell asleep this afternoon. When I woke up I felt fine and for a moment I forgot about everything. Jack was standing over me handing me a tablet.

'What do you think you're doing?' I asked, getting out of bed. I was completely out of it.

I wandered into the kitchen and saw the boys' dinner had been cooked. 'Why are you giving them boiling hot food?' I asked. I grabbed the plates and took them outside to the garden and walked around to cool them down.

Jack was looking at me strangely.

'Jade,' he said, gently. 'Can't you remember anything?'

'What are you talking about?' I asked.

'You've got cancer,' he said. 'You are ill. That's why the bed is downstairs.'

I'd completely forgotten. Isn't that odd? I really lost it for a moment.

Then he had to go because of his curfew.

I've been getting really stressed out about us spending the wedding night together. I so badly want him to be with me. We can't have the reception at Mary's (I had thought about that but there's not enough space) so we had to rely on the probation people changing their minds.

Then today Mark rang me and said something about Jack Straw.

'Who's he?' I said.

'He runs the Justice Ministry,' said Mark. 'He's lifting Jack's curfew so you can spend the wedding night with him.'

I was so happy. What a relief. Thanks to another Jack I get my Jack back!

*   *   *

We had the hen night tonight. We had fake-bake spray tans, dermabrasion, eyebrow threading, nails, feet and eyelash tinting.

Before she slapped it on the beautician asked me if I was sure I was okay with fake bake. 'Chemo treatment can change your skin,' she said. 'So you have to be careful.'

'Yeah, don't worry,' I replied, too excited to listen. Typical me!

I was feeling narky though. I had a bit of a Bridezilla complex. I think I annoyed the girls but it's just because all the wedding stuff was stressing me out. When I noticed that Kel had gone dead quiet, I knew I'd pushed it too far.

'Sorry I'm being so bossy,' I said. 'I'll stop

shouting now.'

I keep forgetting about people I've invited and the list is getting bigger.

'If this mucks up and people can't get in, I will be so embarrassed,' I said. 'Has anyone rung the mums from school and invited them?'

Apparently the bridesmaids didn't have their numbers—what a pathetic excuse!

We ended up with 160 on the guest list. I could have had more but there was no time. Charlene is filming all of this on a camcorder for the TV show. I don't want a real film crew around all the time right now but I don't mind her doing this.

Other people have wedding videos so why not me? Okay, I know mine is a bit unusual, but nothing about my life has ever been normal. Ain't that a fact!

Chapter Nineteen

Here Comes the Bride!

21st February 2009

I woke up screaming—and not with cancer pain this time. There were horrible carrot-coloured patches on my arms, on my tummy, on my legs, all over.

'Arghhhh!' I shrieked.

Kel came rushing in.

'Look at my body, my head, my legs. I look awful,' I screamed.

Someone phoned Victoria Beckham's spray

tannest (is that the right word?) and she agreed to come and sort me out.

Kate turned up. She said she was feeling better now and didn't want to let me down.

She gave me a bath and I kept asking her to scrub my back harder but she didn't like to because she said it is all bony and she doesn't want to hurt me.

I do look fragile now. I don't feel it today, though.

My tube pump thing to pump the drugs in came off my skin and floated in the bath.

I was laughing but Kate was panicking. 'We need the nurse!' she said.

I felt a bit shivery afterwards.

'Why do I keep shivering?' I asked Jen.

'As long as you're not in pain,' she said.

These side effects make me feel so weird.

*   *   *

Kel had picked up some fake bald heads from a joke shop and we all went out to pose for a photo outside my house. The girls didn't half look funny in them.

'See?' I laughed. 'None of you lot can pull it off like me!'

It was touching watching them trying to join in.

Then Simon turned up and we set off to Oxford Street to get our teeth whitened. We headed off in two cars, but Simon got a puncture and had to pull over in a petrol station so five of us all piled into Caroline's mini.

Simon and Charlene got a van from a photographer friend of his and followed behind, like the A-team.

My mouth started to get horribly dry and Simon had the bag with all my drugs so I called him on his mobile and he leapt out in traffic to give me my mouth spray. A few squirts of that sorts me out for a bit.

In the car we talked about what music to play at the wedding.

The song 'Girl so Dangerous' by Akon came on the radio and I started singing along.

'I love this one!' I screamed. 'I want all us girls to dance to this.'

We also wanted a proper band to play.

I wanted Amy Winehouse, as I really love her to bits. I've known Amy's dad Mitch for a few years now. He's a great bloke and said Amy was a fan of mine too.

We rang her agent who considered the idea. Trouble was she was too busy living it up in St. Lucia.

I'd have loved Rod Stewart too, but he was also busy.

Girls Aloud wanted to come but couldn't, then luckily the Sugababes were available.

I've chosen 'I Don't Want to Miss a Thing' by Aerosmith for our first dance because I love the lyrics. And it's true—I don't wanna miss a thing.

Jack thinks it is too sad. 'That one will make everyone cry,' he said.

'Well, that's what I want to happen,' I laughed.

*   *   *

I love getting my teeth whitened. I've always had a thing about clean teeth—that's from my mum. She even used to drag me out of bed at night, insisting

I clean them if I had forgotten. Maybe that's why I became a dental nurse—the job I was doing before I went into the *BB* house.

I made all the girls take pictures of their yellow teeth first. It's amazing how different they turned out after the treatment!

Afterwards we went home and I had a little sleep. I am totally knackered and want to save my energy.

*   *   *

When I woke up, Kev had an idea. He suggested that Jack and I should go out to my driveway and have a little kiss in front of all the paps out there.

'If you go and have a kiss that will make the front page of the papers,' he said, 'Rather than a horrible negative story.'

Jack wasn't too keen. He hates the limelight.

On the way out we started arguing about colours for the ushers. I wanted navy and he was talking about maroon because David Beckham wore it once or something!

We stopped as we reached the drive and saw all the cameras pointing in our direction.

'Hold my face,' I whispered.

So he did. It was a lovely kiss!

*   *   *

My original plan was to fly in to Down Hall by helicopter on the day, but in the end we decided to go the day before because it all got too complicated.

We were due to leave at 4.30pm but Jen and Kel

didn't arrive till 5 and I had the hump by then. I'm so tired. We'd all decided to wear our Pineapple tracksuits. Kate was feeling a bit better, she said, although I later found out that the hospital wanted her to have surgery and she'd refused so she could come to the do. What a star!

I've always loved flying and as the helicopter blades started spinning I got well excited.

'Oooh,' I said, grabbing Jen's hand.

'Can't believe we are doing this,' Jen laughed, and the girls linked arms.

I could feel tears pricking in my eyes and turned to the window.

'I don't want to die,' I said. 'I'll miss all of this.'

'We won't do it without you,' she said, tearfully.

I looked at her. 'Yes, you will,' I said as sternly as I could.

At that moment, the helicopter turned. 'Look,' said Kel. 'Look at your beautiful wedding place down there.'

Down Hall Country House looked amazing, with a marquee set out in the fields behind.

'Oh my god,' I screamed. 'It looks wicked!'

The hotel was gorgeous and our rooms were lush. I lay on my bed and the bridesmaids came in, chatting and looking at the room service menus.

'We should all be jumping up and down on the beds,' I said. 'That's what we'd do if I wasn't ill.'

'It doesn't matter,' said Jen. 'You'll still have the best day ever.'

I am determined to make it the best day ever. Even if I drop dead straight afterwards.

210

22nd February 2009

I woke up in the morning with a familiar sick feeling. Pain was shooting through my sides again. I tried to sit up and groaned. I needed to rest a bit more. I wanted to see everyone but didn't know where they were.

I fell back asleep then woke up to hear a knock at the door.

'We're going to a chapel and we're gonna get maaaaaaaarrrried . . .' sang my bridesmaids as they burst into the room.

My girls know how to make me smile.

We all went downstairs wearing our white towelling hotel robes. We looked so funny.

I had a bowl of fruit to eat.

Of course there was always going to be something to stress me out and this time it was my mum. She'd forgotten to go and get my granddad and nan up, so I sent her off.

Nan came and sat next to me. I buttered her toast. She really needs looking after now.

I had to sign the breakfast bill and Kel was laughing at me for signing 'Mrs Tweed'. I like practising it though.

Then the nurse came to give me my painkillers. I forget I am ill for a second and then—bang!—a reminder. I have a pump that goes into my arm, constantly giving me painkillers, and it needs to be topped up from time to time.

I was excited and happy to be getting married but not really nervous. As Jack says, I don't do nervous!

We had a mammoth make-up session before I got dressed.

I had no energy so said: 'You do whatever you want.'

One by one the bridesmaids came through to me for inspection.

'I hate that silver eyeshadow,' I said. 'Can't you wear blue?'

Caroline, who usually has her hair down, had been given a different sideways style.

The look on her face told me everything.

'You hate it, don't you?' I said.

The girls all laughed. I was right, I knew it.

'Well, at least you have some hair,' I said. I think I made her feel a bit guilty.

I had a go at the girls as they whinged and squabbled about what they wanted.

'You've got the best hair and make-up people here,' I said, 'and you're stressing me out over silly hairstyles.'

I was being narky, but it's my wedding day and I was dying—so it's allowed!

Celebrity hairdresser Richard Ward was doing my mum's hair and I gave her strict instructions to shut up and let him do what he wanted to her. He'd dropped everything for me and he did a fantastic job. Everyone looked great.

Someone had sent me an amazing £10K wig, all brown and straight-styled. I tried it on and the girls whistled at me.

It reminded me of when I used to wear one years ago for a laugh. I thought it looked great on me, and had loads of fun wearing it. I never thought back then that one day I'd be bald and would actually need a wig.

I took it off.

'You know what?' I said. 'I'm bald, everyone

knows I'm bald. And I don't want to be a fake on my wedding day.' So I put it back in the box.

At the end of the day, I am bald now because I'm ill and I can't be bothered with wigs and all that.

Not being full of myself, I think I can carry off this bald look. Loads of people have told me that.

I've got used to it and Jack says I am pretty enough to carry it off.

Some people couldn't. But I can.

*   *   *

Before I got my dress on, I went to make sure everyone else was ready. My nan was sitting in her dressing gown, not doing anything.

'Come on,' I said. 'It's time.'

I knew she was proud of me, and wanted to help her.

Next I gave the boys the posh friendship bracelets I'd bought them.

'Never take them off,' I said. 'And rub them if you're ever sad or missing me and thinking of me.'

Bobby wore his all day. Freddy was a bit young and kept taking it off.

Jack gave me the most gorgeous pre-wedding gift. It was a pair of diamond earrings and a necklace. I gave him a Rolex watch.

*   *   *

I was desperate to get my dress on and go. I knew I only had a limited amount of energy.

'What are we waiting around for?' I asked.

My granddad walked me down the aisle. He was

213

welling up with pride. *I love him so much.*

The bridesmaids came after and looked lovely. I told Kate to go first as she has blonde hair and the others had brown, but she walked a bit fast.

Jack's face was a picture as I arrived. He looked different today somehow. My friends haven't always been Jack's biggest fans but they looked at me and said: 'He seems to have grown into a man today.'

My feet were aching as the bishop read out the vows.

I slipped off my shoes and sat down in the wheelchair and Jack kneeled beside me to look into my eyes.

I got the giggles when Jack read out his lines.

No one touched my life like you. (*You can say that again, Jack!*)

No one can compare to you.

No one made my heart leap and soul jump.

Nor set my mind alight with joy.

In your presence I've found my rest, my home, my self.

In your arms I've found such peace.

Today I give myself to you. I'm yours and ever shall it be.

*   *   *

Then I read my bit out.

You are so handsome to me. (*I couldn't help giggling, but I said 'I mean that!'*)

You are my life, my light, my hope and my joy.

I will treasure you.

I will cherish you.

I will be utterly devoted to you through the laughter and the tears, through the darkness and the light.

I will be your eternal love, your constant companion, your closest friend, pledging to you my deepest commitment and this is my solemn vow.

*   *   *

What with my false eyelashes and my tears, it was any wonder I could see Jack. It was so emotional, I was choked.

My hands were all sticky as we put on the rings.

Then we lit candles as a symbol. The bishop warned me not to spill wax on my dress. I tried my best. The idea is that candles will be lit every anniversary. I hope that helps Jack when I've gone.

The bishop said some really sweet words about my light scattering the darkness and sending it fleeing, which was nice.

He started singing at one point too, which cracked us up. He's a real character.

Kevin did a lovely reading then my friend Roy, who I met while having radiotherapy, gave a reading too. And I don't think there was dry eye in the house.

Just how a wedding should be.

*   *   *

During the official photo shoot, I started to feel pain again. It got so bad I couldn't hold in a moaning sound.

Jen noticed and saw Bobby next to me, his little face full of worry. Being a bit older than Freddy, he notices more about how I am feeling and I could tell he was upset.

215

Jen grabbed his hand and led him away. I heard Mark, Kate and her playing *X Factor* with him as I was given my painkilling jab.

All I could hear was Jen's voice singing his favourite song—'Push the Button'—louder and louder to cover up the noise I was making.

*   *   *

Just before dinner they opened the doors and announced: 'Stand up for Mr and Mrs Tweed.' My heart leapt with excitement.

I am Mrs Tweed!

The food was lovely—duck breast salad, fillet of beef and hazelnut meringue for pud. Gorgeous.

Bobby and Freddy were scoffing the cakes. 'Eat your first course first,' I said.

Richard and Judy leaned over and asked Freddy, 'Are you Bobby?'

'No,' he laughed. 'I'm Freddy. People always say that!'

Max Clifford's wedding present to us was a big surprise. All of a sudden a waitress stood up and made some nervous speech about it being her first wedding at the hotel so she had to . . . then she started singing opera.

Her performance was amazing and it turns out all the staff were full-on singers.

I got into the swing and climbed on my chair at one point to join in. Jack looked a bit embarrassed, but he knows what I'm like! At least, he should do by now.

In his wedding speech Jack said: 'I don't think there's ever been a prouder man standing here tonight. I am proud for what she's achieved in her life and how brave she's been and I'm proud to call her my wife.'

Jack, darling, you did me proud with that speech!

Bobby had written one for me too, then got the jitters and started crying so I read it out.

It said: 'Mummy and Jack, you both look lovely and Mummy you're the best Mummy in the whole wide world and congratulations on your best day ever. Lots of love Bobby and Freddy.'

I was so proud of him. He needed a big cuddle afterwards, though. Bobby can stand up on stage at school no problem but I think he got a bit overwhelmed in front of all the adults.

Granddad stood up next and said: 'I dunno what to say, I've never made a speech in my life. I want to congratulate the happy couple and tell Jade just how much her nan and myself love her. Today when I walked you down the aisle made my life.'

Aw, thanks, Granddad.

Then my best men, Danny and Simon, showed a slide-show of pictures of me and Jack on our holidays. Everyone started crying. Jack's gran was really streaming.

I looked at those pictures of me on jet skis and beaches and they brought back such lovely memories but I felt sad that I won't do all that again. Seeing me up there when I was all healthy was a bit strange. It seems such a long time ago.

I was choked when I read my speech.

I told the bridesmaids how well they've done. 'You are normally so stupid and not with it but you pulled it together. I've had the best of everything—the man who did Elton John's flowers and the best dress, venue and band,' I said. God they did look tired, poor things.

'I love you all so much it makes me not want to leave you,' I said.

The room fell silent as I finished it off. 'In a few years' time, maybe I'll have a blessing and we'll all be here again. So cross your fingers and a miracle might happen.'

You never know. After the day I had it feels like anything is possible.

*　　　*　　　*

We hit the dance floor and Kevin introduced the Sugababes. They were brilliant and I was so glad they could come.

Then Jack and I had our first dance and I couldn't stop snogging him! I still fancy him as much as when we met. I felt so proud as we waltzed around together. It felt like this was always meant to be. I've always dreamed of this day.

Then it was the bridesmaids' dance to 'Girl so Dangerous'. I managed to get down with my heels on, kicking my legs, the lot! I really went for it and so did the girls, just like the old times.

Jack tried a bit of crowd surfing for his ushers' song: 'Apple Bottom Jeans' by T-pain.

Then at 10pm the fireworks were set off. Kel had organised them and I knew she was nervous about it, but in the end they were perfect. As our faces lit up watching the colours, Jack slipped an arm around me and the boys sat on my lap.

Looking round I could see so many people smiling, drinking, laughing. All my closest friends and family. There were hardly any celebs at the do—just Richard and Judy, Aldo Zilli and Jamelia.

I've never felt at home in the celebrity world. Being nice to other famous people just for the sake of it is not my thing. I can truthfully say that every single person in that room meant something to me.

*   *   *

The tiredness I'd been fighting all day started to creep over me. I'd enjoyed a few drinks—champagne and some shots—which probably didn't help. I kissed Jack and said I was going upstairs. Out of all my friends I am usually the one up for the longest, staying till the bitter end. I am the party animal who doesn't know when to stop.

I looked at my bridesmaids all dancing like mad and knocking back the booze. They'd barely eaten for the past week to try and lose some weight for the wedding, so most of them were completely legless.

I felt so proud of them for all they'd achieved that day.

My new husband came upstairs with me and we flopped on the bed. I got out of my dress and then thought I didn't want it to end, so put it back on again. Then I realised I was very tired and flopped back onto the bed.

'Hello, I love you,' Jack said, pecking me on the lips.

We held each other and I felt myself drifting off.

'Go back to the party, Jack,' I said. 'I am too tired to celebrate so do it for both of us. Get the microphone and thank everyone for coming.'

I could tell he felt bad about leaving. But I really didn't mind.

219

He kept popping back to check up on me then I felt a pair of arms wrap around me again about 2am. Jack gave me a beery-smelling kiss, said 'I love you' and then we fell asleep in each other's arms as man and wife.

Mr and Mrs Tweed.

Chapter Twenty

Making Plans

23rd February 2009

I was totally wiped out by yesterday. Today Jack and I spent the day snuggled up naked in the hotel bed, watching TV and relaxing. It was so good to just spend time on our own for once. It might be the only day we ever have together as man and wife. A few close friends and family members popped in to say goodbye.

He told me how he'd gone back to the wedding and spent an hour and a half whizzing round with Bobby on his lap in my wheelchair. I'm glad people can have fun on it. The boys stayed in my mum's room last night.

My fabulous nurses—Isabella, Caroline and Gaynor—popped in from time to time to see if I'm okay. My three shining stars. They are absolutely wonderful.

I've already started to think about the christening. I just keep wanting one more big celebration. I think fancy-dress would be good.

'I'll tell you what,' I said to Jack. 'You can go as

a spoon and I'll go as a boiled egg.'

The look on his face said it all. 'Er, Jade,' he laughed. 'What about something else?' He thought for a second. 'What about Andy and Lou in *Little Britain*? You could go in your wheelchair then.'

It cracked me up.

We sat and opened all our wedding cards and presents. We got some lovely picture frames, vases and a statue of a woman from Richard and Judy.

'Who's this supposed to be?' I asked Jack, holding it out.

'It's probably supposed to be you,' said Jack, smiling.

Danielle gave us a lovely canvas portrait of me, Jack and the kids. That meant a lot to me.

We just got room service sandwiches when we wanted something to eat. I would have liked to stay another night but Jack had to get back home for his curfew, so at 6pm Mary and Jack's sister Laura picked us up.

They packed up the room and stuffed their car with all the presents. Jack sat in the back with his mum, surrounded by flowers. It was like a backseat florist.

My bones started to ache and I got terrible pain suddenly. Laura switched on the heated car seat and it eased a bit.

We chatted about the wedding. 'It was just so great,' I kept repeating.

They dropped me off at my house first before they took Jack home. I didn't want to let my new husband go, but the curfew was back in place.

The wedding was well and truly over. Now I had a christening to plan.

24th February 2009

I watched Kevin and Kel talking about the wedding on *This Morning*. Kel showed her bridesmaid's ring and told them what the engraving said and Kevin showed them the money clip I'd bought him.

Everything that goes out there in the press is checked past me. I don't mind it at all. They can talk for me if they want.

Kate always insists on donating any fees she gets to the boys' fund, even though I told her we can go 50–50. I think she's a mug. Why not make money out of it? But she says it wouldn't feel right.

25th February 2009

My friend Angie, who's been off travelling since December, flew back from Bangkok for four nights to see me. She was shocked at how ill I've got so quickly.

I organised for all the girls to come round for a spag bol, that they would make.

While they were cooking the doorbell rang and it was a package from David and Victoria Beckham containing two football kits. The boys were well excited. They ripped open the packages and soon got into a mess muddling the strips up.

'Come on, boys, sort yourselves out,' I said, trying to wrestle them into order.

Even doing that made me ache.

I used to love taking Bobby for his training at the David Beckham school. I'd watch from the sidelines and imagine him playing for England one day. Jeff was a footballer and although he never made it to the first team, he obviously had talent.

I always say I won't spoil my boys but I can't help it. At least I try and make sure they appreciate everything they have.

The girls had sneaked some pepper into the spag bol and Bobby didn't like it.

'I don't want that, Mum,' he said.

'I knew he'd spot it,' I laughed.

They both made a bit of a mess and got tomato all down their new football shirts.

After dinner, the girls got them in the bath and put them into pyjamas, but I kissed them goodnight before they went to bed.

'We want to play with our Nintendo DS,' said Bobby.

Always the chancer! The night before I'd been up to their room three times and knew I couldn't face that again.

'Listen,' I said. 'If you don't go to sleep the tadpoles in Mummy's tummy won't sleep either.'

They seemed to understand this and went quietly, bless.

When upstairs fell silent I turned to the girls.

'I want to talk to you about my funeral,' I said.

'Don't . . .' began Kelly, welling up.

'I know it's hard, but you need to know. I want my friends to know what I want. It's important.'

They all looked at me, listening. I had to get my words out before anyone cried.

I took a deep breath.

'I want to be buried in my wedding dress,' I said. 'Wearing my wedding rings and with photos of all my family and friends.'

It had been one of the happiest days of my life,

so that seemed right.

I looked at Kelly and Jen. 'You two, I want a reading from you.'

'And I want "Last Request" by Paolo Nutini and "Amazing Grace" because it's Mum's favourite.'

Glancing down, Kelly asked: 'Do you want your boys to come?'

I swallowed, thinking of my two little ones, smartly dressed in black. I tried to push the image out of my head.

'I . . . I don't know. I think they're too young. What do you think?'

I turned to Angie. Her mum had died when she was little.

'Did you go?' I asked her.

She shook her head.

'Did you regret not going?'

'No,' she replied.

'Then maybe they won't either then.' I said.

I still haven't told them I won't be around for long. Of course, it's a conversation no mother wants to have. I've got that book *Badger's Parting Gift* that explains death to young kids. The hospital will tell me when it's time to read it.

* * *

Bobby wakened up and wanted to get out of his own bed and sleep in my empty double bed. Instead I went and got him and gave him a piggyback downstairs to my hospital bed.

We slept top to tail. It was so lovely to feel his soft warm skin against mine. He felt so safe and happy lying there with his mum. And he won't enjoy this feeling for much longer. *My poor babies.*

224

I can't drive them to school any more because my medication is affecting my eyesight. It breaks my heart to think I'll never do that again.

It breaks my heart that I won't see them growing up. I can't think about any of that. I mustn't. It's just too much.

Chapter Twenty-one

Hanging in There

26th February 2009

The pain was so terrible I could hardly sleep. I just rolled from side to side, feeling like I'd do anything to escape it, but trying not to make a sound in case I wakened Bobby. Usually when you cry tears you feel better. With this kind of pain nothing works.

When I woke up Bobby had already got up and I started screaming and crying because I didn't know where I was or why there were people in my house. The nurse explained gently that the drugs are making me hallucinate. It was terrifying. I'm taking a new drug and it's made me go mental. I just wanted Jack to stay by me.

My doctors said I need to go to St Clare's hospice in Harlow to change my medicine. I don't want my boys to see their mum in this terrible state, no way. I wanted to go to the Marsden because they can always control the pain better. I feel safer there. They know what they're doing with cancer pain. But they said the hospice will do just as good a job and they're much closer.

*   *   *

Jack came round and I told him again he can have the house if he wants. He looked at me and shook his head. 'I'd just be looking for you in every corner,' he said.

I feel like I want to protect him. What is he going to do after I've gone?

I suggested maybe he should take half the money from the wedding. He looked shocked. 'I don't want that,' he said. 'It's for the boys.'

He's got to take the Rolex watch I bought him to the jewellers'. His wrists are so skinny, it's too big for him.

27th February 2009

I managed to get dressed to go in the car to go to St Clare's hospice.

As Jack helped me into the car, all the paps started snapping like crazy. My old neighbour, who was washing his car, started tutting and making comments. I don't know what he was saying but he really wound me up. I feel so weepy anyway, his dirty looks got right up my nose.

I think it had something to do with the paps blocking our narrow lane. It wasn't affecting him that much. The road was big enough for everyone to share.

I could see he was still pissed off.

'Leave me alone!' I screamed at him as Jack opened the car door. 'I'll be dead in a month anyway!'

All the paps went crazy, scrabbling for a picture.

Why is he acting like this? He can have his peace and quiet after I've gone.

We drove off really fast, and I was in tears all the way. Even going out of my front door has to be a drama.

*   *   *

I'm not sure how long I'll be in the hospice so I asked Mum to bring me my photos of the boys, some DVDs, crisps, chocolate, cake and sweets.

The pain got really bad. It wasn't my cancer pain this time—it was my bowels all blocked again as I can't go to the toilet.

It's so stupid to be in pain because of this. I couldn't believe no one could just give me something. I asked the nurses for an extra-big suppository. Fingers crossed that will work.

*   *   *

Charlene stayed over at the hospice with me and I told her I want to start planning the christening now. I got the laptop and we started looking things up.

I've decided I want a marquee, a kids' entertainer, an ice-cream van, candyfloss, face paints and animals for the kids. We tried ringing a few companies but we only got their answerphones because it was the evening and they'd closed. I called Mark and told him to get going on it.

I've decided on fancy-dress outfits too. I chose a showgirl outfit for myself (like in a Broadway musical such as *Chicago*) and Charleston girl outfits for the bridesmaids. Everyone else can come as they want.

'You do know we have to be in a church?' Charlene asked.

'Yeah, yeah,' I replied. 'I'm sure they won't mind.'

The news got out that I am hoping to do a last interview with Piers Morgan. He approached asking if I could do it but I'm not sure if I'm going to be well enough.

Apparently my dad's mum, Jacqueline Goody, wants to get back in touch. She was a druggie too. I never had much to do with her and to be honest I don't even know her. It's not going to happen.

There's so little time left. I have to keep it all for my loved ones now.

28th February 2009

It was Jen's birthday on the 26th and she wanted me to go out for lunch today but I am too ill.

Wendy Richards, who played Pauline in *EastEnders*, has died of cancer. It's weird watching what happens on TV when people die. Everyone is upset and saying nice things about her. I hope they do that about me.

I didn't know Wendy personally—even though the papers claimed we met at the Marsden—but I felt a bit sad anyway. I hope she didn't suffer too much in the end. *I hope I don't either.*

Someone told me that apricot kernels can cure cancer so I've been trying to eat as many as I can. Unfortunately they taste vile!

Found out today I was voted the third most respected person in the world in an internet poll, Onepoll.com. I'm just behind Barack Obama and Nelson Mandela! Can you believe it? I was genuinely moved.

I felt a bit better later and Jen's mum, Sue, came to see me. She brought cod, chips and curry sauce and we talked about old times. I love Jen's mum.

Apparently Larry King and Oprah Winfrey in America want to interview me now. I'd never heard of Larry King until Mark told me who he was. It's just not going to happen—sadly, as I'd love the money for Bobby and Freddy.

I've got a couple more money-making plans still. Kate is going to bring out a limited-edition perfume and Danny will organise a picture tribute book, all proceeds to go to the boys' fund. And then *OK!* will pay to cover the christening. Every bit helps.

1st March 2009

Going back to the Marsden today. I asked for Matt, the ambulanceman I've used before, because we really get on. I asked him about his children. He held my hand and I told him what a good man he is. Then the pain was really bad again and he gave me gas and air. I went a bit woozy and lovely, like I'd had a G&T. It didn't last though.

It was weird in the ambulance, all neon blue and flashing lights. It took ages to get there. There was a police convoy with us and they shut the M11. I can't believe just how big this has got.

When we got to the hospital, the pain was so bad I begged the doctors to give me a colostomy bag—anything to stop it, anything.

I had to have an examination and asked Kate to hold my hand because it's so uncomfortable. Apparently I need a procedure but I don't care even if they open me up.

'If I have to die, don't let this pain last until then,' I screamed at them.

I had an X-ray about 4pm. Afterwards I was still in so much pain, I couldn't bear it.

'Stop this!' I screamed. 'Please get them to give me something, anything, please!' I grabbed Kate's collar and cried in her face.

The doctors have this 'pain scale' and asked me how bad it was from one to ten.

'Ten! Ten!' I screamed.

They all started trying to sort out the medicines but they take a while to work.

My skin is flaking and scabby. I feel disgusting. I can't live like this. Kate told me she could put some moisturiser on for me but that's not the point, she doesn't understand. It's going to take more than a bit of make-up to sort this out.

My body is horrible now. I don't want to be like this.

Finally the drugs kicked in and I felt calmer. I spent an hour chatting to Danny and Kate. I told them I wasn't religious but I've always believed in God. I am wearing a cross someone sent me, tied up with Jack's tracksuit cord.

I am so worried about Jack. Where is he going to live? I want him to sell his story so he can put a deposit on a flat, but he still says that all the money should go to the boys.

Someone sent in a massive fruit basket and I had some strawberries with chocolate on. I threw a bit in the bin and Kate said she'd eat it so as not to waste it.

'You can't,' I said. 'My mouth is all scabby.' I'm worried I might give her something with all the white yuck on my tongue.

I talked to Danny about the picture book I want him to do.

'I want my boys to remember me,' I said. 'Make sure you help them so they don't forget.'

He got out his laptop and we went through a few pictures. I told him I don't want any of me lying on a stretcher.

'Hey, you should do some fun ones of me now,' I giggled. 'Get that bow and make me look like an Easter egg.'

Danny took the bow off the fruit basket and put it on my head so I looked like a big baby.

'Coochee coochee coooo,' they laughed, taking pictures.

I tried to push Kate out of the shot. 'You're always trying to steal the limelight,' I joked.

2nd March 2009

It was bad again last night. My tummy is killing me.

I'm being transferred to the Chelsea and Westminster hospital for a procedure on my bowel. They have to do the mini op there because it's a special one. There is a blockage and they need to do a bypass. My body just feels like one big organ now. Not something that belongs to me, just a failing machine doctors keep poking at. A young person's body that feels old and doesn't work.

Thankfully the op got the pain sorted. I told them it's gone down from a ten to a six. Such relief!

I woke up very woozy. Can't speak much and keep drifting off.

*   *   *

Kate turned up and I told her to go away and then I screamed at her to get me another pillow.

Charlene also showed up and I asked her why she'd come.

'Oh, now you're here just get me some toothpaste and a toothbrush please,' I said.

'It's 9.30pm . . . where . . .?' she started, then rushed off to find one.

They are good to me.

3rd March 2009

Jack got special permission to stay with me last night, which was lovely, but he had to go to court this morning. He's had his second brush with the law. I didn't read all the gory details and didn't ask him about it—am in too much pain—but I heard later he has been convicted for assaulting a cabbie and will be sentenced on the 14th of April.

I've tried not to hear about it. What's important is that he's been there for me—yes, despite all the pap shots of him being out with his mates. I tell him to go out sometimes. He's a young guy who shouldn't be stuck in a hospital 24/7 and, besides, I

232

need to rest.

Most of the time he is with me anyway. He buys me presents, like a lovely new outfit from Zara and some underwear to cheer me up. It means so much to me when people do normal things.

'I just wish I could be here all the time,' he said last night, stroking my cheek. 'I am so sorry for my behaviour and not being here all the time. I know I have let you and everyone down.'

He made me well up again. I know he is sorry. He gets such a bad press, but really he is amazing to me. He is the one person who makes me feel complete.

No one should forget how hard this is on him. It's horrible to see someone you love in so much pain. I can't believe I ever doubted his ability to cope.

4th March 2009

Just feel really weak. Have hardly spoken because I slept for most of the day. When I come round Jack is usually holding my hand. He looks after me so well. He's great at cleaning my teeth, washing me, helping me to the loo. I only really want and need him. I tried to speak to him about what will happen after I'm gone but he hates talking about it.

'I want you to make as much money out of the magazines as possible,' I said. 'Do it while you can. Then buy a flat so the boys can come and stay over any time. So they don't forget me.'

'But I don't want to use your fame for money like that,' he said. 'I don't want to live off someone else.'

'Then do it for the boys,' I said. 'And I want you meet someone nice . . .'

Jack looked horrified. 'I don't want anyone else,' he said.

I smiled. 'You are not going to stay single for the rest of your life.'

'It's up to me,' he said. 'It's my life, Jade.'

I pushed him and he admitted that maybe he would meet someone, one day.

'But what if she doesn't like my boys seeing you?' I asked.

'Then I won't be with her,' said Jack.

'Jack, you know I will still be here though, don't you? You know when you look up at night, at the sky, I will be the biggest star you've ever seen?'

'You've always been the biggest star to me,' he said.

I told him a few of the songs I want for my funeral.

'I don't want to talk about it,' said Jack, looking really upset.

'Okay, I'll tell someone else,' I said.

I thought about my plans to make a video for the boys. With the wedding and everything it never happened. I can't see that I'll be able to do it now.

Chapter Twenty-two

The Last Journey

5th March 2009

I put in a request today to the hospital chaplain to get christened with the boys as soon as we can. I possibly only have a few days. It's the only way I can make sure I'll go to Heaven and the boys can reach me through Jesus. I really want to go to Heaven. I want to find some kind of peace.

I told the boys today that the tadpoles are getting stronger and I might have to go to Heaven soon.

They are keeping to their normal routine as much as possible, going to school, seeing their dad. Kids need routine. I don't want them to know the ins and outs. They are too young.

Jeff told me that Bobby told his schoolmates, 'My mummy is going to Heaven.'

Later Freddy got two chocolate tractors and gave Jack one and said to save the other for me when I get to Heaven. He doesn't understand what's happening at all.

I called Kate. 'I've only got a couple of days left now,' I said to her.

They've not directly told me but I know. I know we have to hurry this christening up. Called Danny and my Mum and told them.

Kate stayed overnight in the day room with Danny. The nurse told them they could if they wanted to. I think they were scared I was going to die in the night.

6th March 2009

When I woke up I saw Kate and Danny standing over my bed. Danny was in a right state. He'd been sick and looked pale and tired.

I couldn't help smiling. 'You should go home,' I said. 'You'll stink after sleeping here.'

They didn't want to leave me but I said I'd be fine. I had my laptop and wanted to choose stuff for the christening now.

*   *   *

The girls all trooped into my room later. I was half asleep, as usual. I felt so weak I couldn't even sit up.

They looked lovely—hair done nicely, make-up, smiling. I knew I looked awful. I feel awful. I hate my friends and the people I love seeing me like this.

'We've just come in for a few minutes to say hello,' said Kelly, gently.

I opened my mouth to speak. My tongue felt all thick and hard.

Such sadness built up inside me it was like my heart was breaking.

'I don't want you girls to come any more,' I said, slowly, and their eyes filled up. 'It breaks my heart to see you.'

7th March 2009

This morning we got christened in the chapel at the Royal Marsden at 11.30am. I had wanted a huge party with a bouncy castle and bumper cars—a kids' paradise. In the end there just wasn't time and the doctors said I was too weak.

It will be covered by a magazine to make more money for the boys. After this I won't be doing any more media work. This is it. Things are too hard now.

Caroline had ordered loads of flowers but we couldn't use them as you're not allowed them in the hospital.

I had an epidural in the morning to control my pain for the ceremony but it meant my legs were numb and not working. I wanted to walk, but there was no way. I arrived after everyone else, in a wheelchair, wearing my hospital gown and slippers. For some people it was the first time they'd seen me since I'd got married. I knew I looked a lot worse.

I insisted on getting out of the wheelchair and sitting in a pew at least.

It wasn't quite what I had in mind and was very sad but lovely at the same time.

As soon as we got in the room, the boys were off pointing at the stained-glass window and climbing in the pews. Freddy started to clamber all over the organ at one point. Mr Nosy! I could only watch them. I use all my energy just to sit upright.

It fills my heart with such sadness that I can't keep up with them.

Jeff told me later that Bobby asked: 'Is Mummy going to wear a wedding dress today?'

He said: 'Not this time. She is going to be baptised and so are you.'

I'd always wanted to get the boys christened and never got round to it. Jeff and I split up just before Freddy was born, so there was too much going on.

It's my way of feeling closer to Bobby and Freddy when I'm gone and for them to feel closer to me. I want them to believe in God and Heaven so they know I am in a good place, waiting for them. I want them to know I am safe and looking over them and that when you die you don't just stop living. You end up somewhere else.

I know I look frail now, but I tried to keep the smiles coming when I could. I can't speak much.

Corinne Brixton, vicar of St John's Church in Buckhurst Hill, near where Jack lives, did the service. She told us how the water washed away our sins and brought us closer to God.

Then there was a reading from the *Good News Book of Romans*.

Bobby was a bit nervous of the water and started crying, bless him! (Well, quite literally.)

I've been reading the Bible more since I've been ill, yet I've always believed in God. I raised my head as the vicar did the cross sign on me too. I felt so peaceful and pleased I'd made it.

Everyone clapped and then someone took a family picture with Jeff, the boys, Jack and me. I leaned into Jack's shoulder just as the camera snapped.

It's good for the boys to see us together. I want Jack to keep in touch with them. Jeff knows he is good with them so I hope he'll let him.

The nurses insisted I get back in my wheelchair. They are so kind to me. I feel so loved by them too.

As they pushed me away, I said: 'Please stop at every pew.'

I just wanted to say goodbye and thanks.

Everyone leant forward one by one and kissed my cheek.

My voice came out all croaky.

I couldn't see some people because my eyes were so blurred. I rubbed them with frustration.

As we reached the doorway I raised my hand to say goodbye.

I don't know when I'll see some of these people again. Or if.

8th March 2009

I woke up today to find a security man in my room and I heard voices and panic.

Jack later explained a woman had got into my room. She was holding a hammer and saying a prayer.

'What did she want?' I asked.

'Just to make you better,' said Jack. 'She was a bit of a nutter.'

Security took her away. I felt sorry for her but was too tired to notice, to be honest.

Jack says the papers are full of my story. It must be hard for my family and friends reading about it. I want to make sure that none of my closest friends hear about me dying from the press. Someone has to make sure they all get a phone call from one of us.

9th March 2009

Just been drifting in and out again. Tiredness keeps taking over. Even sipping on my drinks takes it out of me.

So many people are wishing me well. Mary said a lady who she didn't know from a bar of soap turned up on her doorstep asking if they could pray together. Mary, being nice, didn't want to let her in but joined her in a prayer outside.

A member of the public sent us three lovely glass angels—one for me, Bobby and Freddy. They are so sweet. I stared at them for ages.

10th March 2009

Today Jack was taught how to help give me painkilling shots of morphine.

This afternoon he popped out for some fresh air and my mum said, 'It's time for your injections, Jade.'

'Where's Jack?' I asked. 'I want him because I don't want the nurses to do it.'

Mum smiled. 'That's good. You can still order us around then,' she said.

Katie Price has been in touch and says she'll fly over from America to see me. It's sweet of her but I don't think there would be much to say.

Robbie Williams sent me some flowers too and I don't even know him! Mum says she put them in the living room.

My vision is getting more blurry now. Something to do with the drugs.

Jack spoke to Michael Jackson today when I was

asleep. Apparently he was trying to get hold of me but people thought it was a wind-up. Somehow he got Jack's number.

He repeated the conversation to me:

'Hello, it's Michael Jackson.'

'Alright, mate.'

'I just want to send Jade my love and positive thoughts.'

'She thinks you're a bit of a legend.'

'I really want her to come to the summer shows.'

'She'd love that, I'll pass it on.'

Later on one of his entourage sent a mobile phone with a message recorded on it. It said: 'Hello Jade, It's Michael Jackson. I want you to know how much I love you and am thinking of you. You need to have positive thoughts as I so want you to come to my show in the summer. Just focus on the good not the bad and we love you, Jade, and will see you in the summer.'

Jack was well impressed and transferred it to his mobile phone to keep.

Funny how all these famous people are wishing me well. Nice of them to take the time.

*   *   *

This evening I watched the rough cut of my wedding on DVD. I'd told Kate I was worried that I might not live to see my own wedding on TV so she sorted out a tape double quick. I cuddled the boys on my lap as we watched it.

It was lovely seeing it. Like reliving the day.

The bishop said that I was laughing in the face of death and it was a privilege to be part of it. Ahhhhh! The boys looked so cute as well. I am *so so* glad we did it.

The only thing that annoyed me was Kate walking too fast down that aisle and I told her so! Still the bossy bride!

I've had my big day and that's made me happy.

11th March 2009

I went home in an ambulance today. Jack held my hand all the way. The probation people say he can spend the night at my house tonight, thank God.

I could hardly see straight as a photographer took a picture.

We have Marie Curie nurses staying with us. One has been doing this job for thirty years!

Now I am so ill, I can't talk very much. I slur a bit, so I spend most of my time listening.

My husband is so lovely to me. I sleep most of the time, but he cares for me very gently.

He cleans my teeth, changes my underwear, washes me gently with a flannel.

Despite all of what is happening, he knows I want to be clean and neat.

The nurse showed him how to lift me gently. I could feel him putting his hands under my arms so lightly. I feel all bony now, but he didn't hurt me at all.

The nurse nodded as he did it. Her eyes filled up and she went into the kitchen to see Mary.

When she returned, she said to him: 'In all my time as a nurse I have never seen a man look after his wife so beautifully. I just had to tell your mum how proud she should be.'

I looked at her and smiled, unable to get my

words out. But inside my head I was saying: 'I am proud of him too.'

The curfew rules have changed and he can stay here on Thursday and Saturday nights now. *I wonder how many nights we have left? All the days are blurring into one.*

*   *   *

I don't know what's going to happen. I do know that my body will slowly stop working and it makes me so sad to think I am just lying here waiting.

I started to feel scared again at how long this is going to take.

I had a bit of a weep with Mum. 'Can you make it happen quicker?' I asked. 'Let them give me an injection.'

Mum bit her lips, trying hard not to cry. 'I'll speak to the nurse,' she said.

When I woke up later, Mum was holding my hand. 'You know what you were saying?' she said. 'The nurse says if we gave you something you could have a heart attack and that wouldn't be nice, would it? If we wait for things to happen slowly your organs will close down and you'll just drift off in your sleep.'

I nodded. I trust my mum, Jack and the nurses to make this as easy as possible.

Not easy, but less bad.

12th March 2009

People think when you're dying you can't eat. I still have my appetite, though. I love chicken, lettuce and mayo sandwiches and bits of chocolate.

I love my fizzy drinks too. This lunchtime I cracked open a can and started glugging it down.

Then Mum came into the room and told me off! 'Stop gulping it,' she said. 'You've got to sip it or you'll get hiccups and that wouldn't be good.'

'Why?' I asked.

'Because the nurse told me it could give you heart attack!'

Apparently because my heart is beating really hard to keep my body alive now, it's more sensitive and hiccups could harm me.

Ice-cream goes down a treat. It's easy to eat and takes away any nasty tastes in my mouth.

This afternoon the boys came in from school, all excited to see me, but Bobby looked shy and hung back. I could only hold his hand. My brave little soldier can't deal with this.

'Hello, Mummy,' he said, and I knew he was upset. It's confusing for the boys because ages ago we told them my hair would grow back when I got better. And it is growing back now but I am not getting better.

Bobby showed me his book and whispered something.

'Speak loudly, Bobby,' said Mum. 'Otherwise she won't hear you and she gets frustrated.'

'Our table at school got a gold medal for good writing,' he said. I started clapping but my hands missed each other.

Mum burst out laughing. 'Did you see that, Bobby? Mummy missed her hands.'

He started giggling too.

Freddy is less self-conscious and threw his arms around me, and lay on my chest.

'Mummy, I don't want you to go to Heaven,' he said, looking me in the eye. 'How will I see or speak to you?'

I felt really calm and my words came out slowly. 'You know how Nanna always thinks of a bumblebee as her granddad who died?' I said. 'Well, every time you see an angel you must think of me.'

'But where do I see angels, Mum?' asked Freddy.

'They will be all around you,' I said. 'In the sky, everywhere.'

'Can you tell them I don't want to have to wait for very long,' he replied.

Mum made dinner tonight. The boys had salmon and veg. I just had ice-cream as I'd already eaten earlier today.

Jack stayed over again as the probation people have fitted a tag machine in my house now. But he can still only stay on Thursdays and Saturdays.

Jack, Kel and Charlene all sat and watched the wedding DVD but I stayed in bed.

Kate popped in and gave me a kiss. Everything is a big effort now, words are hard. She kissed me on my head and told me she loved me. I managed to blow her one back.

13th March 2009

I keep drifting off. Can hardly keep my eyes open. People are in and out all day. Granddad held my hand for an hour, bless him. I hate to think of him upset. I know it's so hard for them.

My nan, who has Alzheimer's, sat with me too.

245

She seemed a lot better today and I think she understood everything that was going on.

My mum is in and out all day long. She's lost a lot of weight, down from eight and a half to seven stone. She looks gaunt, like she did in her drug days. My poor mum.

Kevin sits with me for a few minutes every day, holding my hand, kissing my cheek.

It's hard for him too.

'You know I am going to a better place, Kev,' I smiled.

'I know you are,' he replied. 'I am not even christened but you make me feel like I'm going there too.'

Of course the person I can stay awake for longest is Jack. Every single second is precious. I stayed awake for two and half hours today.

Jack and his friend Jasper have been opening my post for me. Some people just write 'Jade Goody Tweed, Essex' on the envelope and it gets to me. I've had so many things sent in.

A week ago we only had a few bottles of holy water, but now it's into the gallons! I've got hundreds of rosary beads. Someone sent in £15 in notes. I think all these people are so kind, taking the trouble.

I told Mum I really fancy West Indian food tonight. The boys are spending the weekend with Jeff. They are going to the *X Factor* show with him. But I know they'll come straight back if they need to.

14th March 2009

I've just been drifting off to sleep. Find it hard to stay awake now.

Jack is here, always here. He holds my hand and we just sit together.

Mum said the boys had superglued a one-pound coin outside the front door to trick her, but she saw them doing it.

Jack's sister Laura came and read out a letter from the Queen's secretary. 'I have been instructed to convey the Queen's warmest good wishes to Jade at what must be a very difficult time for her and her family.'

Laura had written to her asking for her support because she knows how much I love the Queen.

I couldn't say much. I just smiled. 'The Queen,' I said. That was so nice.

15th March 2009

Only Mum and Jack and the nurses are here now. I heard Mum say 'only close family and friends'. I think Kevin is still hanging around too.

I just sleep.

Jack hardly leaves my side. I can see it's a sunny day through the blinds. They are all half-closed, but I can see the fields through my window. I managed to sip cans of Coke and Fanta.

'The boys are on their way,' Jack whispered.

I so wanted to see them, I don't want them to see me like this, though.

Bobby and Freddy came in with Jeff, holding daffodils. They'd been playing outside in the sun in the garden. I could hear them shouting and laughing.

Then they went all quiet as they came inside. Jeff looked emotional when he dropped them off.

Their faces had been painted. Bobby's was all black—I'm not sure what he was supposed to be— and Freddy was a tiger. They came in to watch their *Toy Story* DVD with me. We lay and had a cuddle and I drifted off for a bit, then when I woke up I realised Bobby was asleep as well. It was a lovely, close, special moment.

Freddy looked at me and smiled, holding my hand.

'Why are you so sleepy, Mummy?' he asked.

I opened my mouth to speak. It takes so much effort. 'Because the angels are calling Mummy now,' I said.

'I don't want you to go to Heaven,' he said. 'I am going to stay at my friend Knick-nack's house tonight and I want Nanna to ring me and tell me if you're Jade Mummy or Jade Heaven.'

When it was time for them to go they both kissed me on the cheek and said goodbye. I said 'I love you' to both of them and they both replied: 'Love you, Mummy.'

I hope they can pop back after school one day next week. I'm so very tired. Just seeing them for a few minutes took all of my energy. *I love them so much.*

My Daughter's Last Days

by Jackiey Budden

16th March 2009

Jade hardly woke up at all today and the nurses say she is nearing the end. But they've been saying that for a while.

A bunch of tulips was delivered to the door with a note that said: 'Thank you for giving us Jade. God must need an angel to make Heaven smile.'

I heard voices in the room and went in to find Jack there.

'She just called me "Jeff"!' he said sadly.

'This is your husband . . .' I told her.

'He was until 30 seconds ago,' she said.

I looked at Jack questioningly.

'She thinks I haven't got the right football kit for the boys,' he explained.

'We'll make sure we get the right ones,' I reassured her and she closed her eyes and drifted into sleep.

She wakened briefly later on while I was sitting holding her hand. 'I don't want to come back as a bumblebee like your granddad,' she said. 'Knowing my luck I'd get swatted.'

I can't believe she can still make jokes. My beautiful daughter is still in there. Her spirit's still strong even if her body is slowly shutting down.

This morning Jade told Jack that she doesn't want the boys to see her die.

'That's not going to happen,' he reassured her.

We take turns reading her bits from the Bible because it seems to make her calm. Charlene has been staying here and when she read out a verse that says 'Call to me and I'll answer . . .' Jade suddenly opened her eyes and spoke. 'I want the bridesmaids to get a tattoo of that. Will they do it?'

'Of course we will,' Charlene said.

'I want one too. Mum, will you call the tattoo man?'

How can I tell her it's too late? It can't be done now.

'Look, I'll get one instead,' I promised. That seemed to calm her down and she drifted off again.

*   *   *

Margo, one of the Marie Curie nurses, is Irish. She'd brought some four-leaved-clover green glasses that morning for St. Patrick's Day and I was wearing them when I went into the room.

'Top of the morning to you,' Jade said, in her best Irish accent. Unbelievable that she can still do that. She was always wicked at accents.

'Can you see my glasses?' I asked her. I wasn't sure how far she could see any more.

'Yes, I can, Mum. Now take them off 'cos they look stupid and you're talking bollocks,' my beautiful daughter said to me.

18th March 2009

This morning I sat and told Jade that the boys will have all her DVDs to watch as they grow up. All her fitness videos and every single documentary she's ever done. 'They can see every point of your life from 2002 onwards,' I told her. 'They will never forget you.'

Later on I told her I was popping out to the shops. I'd got halfway down the road when one of the nurses came rushing after me to say she was calling for me, so I turned and ran back up to the house.

'Thought you were going to the shops,' Jade said when I came in the room.

'I was! I rushed back because you called.'

'Oh,' she said. 'Sorry.'

Then she fell asleep again.

Later, she woke up and thought she was looking after a newborn baby. She cradled it in her arms for a while then called Jack.

'Jack, can you take this baby for me?' she asked. 'He's called Simon.'

Jack pretended to take a baby from her and give it a cuddle.

'Will you look after him?' she asked, and Jack said he would.

'Good,' she said. 'I can go to sleep now.'

19th March 2009

This morning Jade woke up and told Jack she needed the loo. He didn't know whether to get the

251

toilet or a bedpan.

'Does it make a difference?' she said. 'I am going to die in about ten minutes anyway.'

Later on we tried showing her some pictures to see who she recognised in them.

'Do you know who this is?' I asked, holding one up.

'It's me, Jack, Bobby and Freddy,' she said. 'I am not a fucking idiot.'

She's still in there, still fighting. It breaks my heart into a million pieces thinking about the enormity of what I'm going to lose.

20th March 2009

Memories from long ago were coming into Jade's mind today.

'Did you know pineapples make you a million pounds?' she said to Jack.

He didn't have a clue what she was talking about.

'You know, Mum,' she said. 'You remember that home help and the pineapples?'

When Jade was seven we had a home help who bought pineapples for me. Except that they weren't on my shopping list and I didn't want or need them! So when she came back for the money I didn't want to pay for them. What a strange thing for Jade to be thinking about.

'All your old memories are coming back,' I told her. 'Isn't that funny?'

She closed her eyes and went back to sleep again.

They said her kidneys would be packing up soon

252

but she can still use the loo so I guess they're still working. She takes tiny sips of Coke or Fanta when she's awake.

She told me she wants to donate her organs and I said I would find out about it. Her heart is strong, she says. And someone can have her eyes. Her lovely eyes.

The boys are going to come back for Mother's Day on Sunday. I told Jade I'll do a picnic for them then.

21st March 2009

Jade didn't waken all day today. Her breathing got fainter and fainter. And then she died at 3.14am on Mothering Sunday, the 22nd of March, as I held her hand.

Epilogue

by Jackiey Budden

My beautiful daughter has gone.

It broke our hearts to let her go, but it was also terrible to watch her worsening every day. She was so strong to the end, defying the doctors who believed she would pass away the weekend before.

In many ways we were glad she'd finally found her peace. She is out of that terrible pain now.

Words aren't enough to express just how proud I am of Jade.

In the end she touched so many lives. The piles of bouquets and some 70,000-plus letters prove how much she meant to so many.

I was proud of her before her illness and feel even more so now.

Jade showed the world how to have a laugh, and that it doesn't matter where you come from—it only matters where you end up. Not only did she make people smile but she also showed them how to die with humour, love, bravery and dignity.

Through her wedding and her love for Jack and the boys she proved that the only thing that really matters in life is love.

I don't know how I will cope without her. I will just try and learn from her strength to be the best Nanna ever for those two boys. She knows I will do my best for them. They will need me now that she has gone.

Jade is a proper star. She was my star and, as she said before she died, she will be the biggest star in the sky up there.

My little girl achieved more in the last seven years than most people will do in a lifetime. She's made more women than ever aware of the horrors of cervical cancer and will probably save countless lives.

The whole wide world will be a sadder place without her, but a better place for her once having been here.

Jade was a Goody in every sense of the word. I love you, Jade. Find your peace now.

Mum X

Jade's Wish List

1. For Bobby and Freddy to visit a Third-World country and do things like make mud huts. I want them to realise that they are very lucky boys and not everyone is as lucky as them.
2. I want them both to have a Porsche as their first car. I got Bobby a little mini Porsche for his first birthday and I've had the idea ever since.
3. I'd like them to go to university and the money is there if they want to. If they don't want to they don't have to.
4. I want them to stay close to my mum Jackiey and Jack. I'd love Jack to take them on the school runs sometimes.
5. I'd like my boys to have good jobs that pay a lot of money. I'd like Bobby to be a lawyer or a footballer, maybe, like David Beckham. Freddy could be a racing car driver.
6. I want both boys to live in one of my houses if they want to. I have a four-bed house in Ongar with a hot tub and a three-bed house in Harlow. They can decide between themselves who lives in what.
7. I don't want my boys to mess the girls around (although I have a feeling they will). Bobby will be a heartbreaker, I can see it. Freddy will definitely mess with girls. Both my sons are the best-looking children, but I hope they are good too!
8. I want both boys to carry on eating really well. I always say finish your plate before you go and play. I want them to carry on eating proper

dinners, like home-made shepherds' pie, spag bol, and good breakfasts like scrambled egg on toast.

9. Holidays and travel. I want the boys to go away and visit lots of places, just as I have.

Acknowledgements

All the royalties of this book will go to Jade's boys, Bobby and Freddy.

Thank you to everyone who has helped and contributed to the diaries: mum Jackiey Budden; husband Jack Tweed; the bridesmaids—Kate, Kel, Jen, Caroline and Charlene; Jade's best men Danny Hayward and Simon Bridger; the Tweed family; Danielle; grandparents John and Sylvie; Dr Ann Coxon; Gill Paul; *OK!* magazine; and *New!* magazine.

And a final thanks to Shannon Kyle and Mark Thomas for helping to pull Jade's diaries together, as Jade would have wanted.

From the Trustees